MW01109261

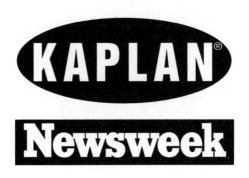

Medical School Admissions Adviser 2001

SELECTION • ADMISSIONS • FINANCIAL AID

by Maria Lofftus and Thomas C. Taylor
with a nationwide team
of medical school admissions advisers

Simon & Schuster

NEW YORK · LONDON · SINGAPORE · SYDNEY · TORONTO

Kaplan Books
Published by Simon & Schuster
1230 Avenue of the Americas
New York, NY 10020

For bulk sales to schools, colleges, and universities, please contact: Order Department, Simon & Schuster, 100 Front Street, Riverside, NJ 08075. Phone: 1-800-223-2336. Fax: 1-800-943-9831.

Project Editor: Ruth Baygell
Cover Design: Cheung Tai
Interior Production: Amparo Graf
Desktop Publishing Manager: Michael Shevlin
Production Editor: Maude Spekes
Managing Editor: Dave Chipps
Executive Editor: Del Franz

Special thanks to: Amy Baxter, Mike Cantwell, William Dracos, Andy Koh, Kiernan McGuire, Susan Pace, Michael Syptak, M.D., and Sara Pearl.

Manufactured in the United States of America
Published simultaneously in Canada

July 2000
10 9 8 7 6 5 4 3 2 1

ISBN: 0-684-87336-2
ISSN: 1097-5411

CONTENTS

Part Six: FINANCING YOUR DEGREE

Appendixes: MEDICAL SCHOOLS

AUTHORS

Maria Lofftus was recently Kaplan's director of academic services for the health sciences. Prior to that she was assistant dean for admissions at the University of California at San Diego, School of Medicine. During her nineteen years in medical school admissions, Ms. Lofftus held numerous leadership positions within the Association of American Medical Colleges, including serving as a member of the Committee for the Expanded Minority Admissions Exercise, as a trainer-facilitator for the Expanded Minority Admissions Exercise, and as chair of the Committee on Admissions. Currently she is the vice president of sales and marketing at nschool.com, a leading K–12 teacher-driven communications service.

Thomas C. Taylor joined the Kaplan team as associate director of academic services for the health sciences in October 1998. Prior to that he was director of admissions and associate director of student affairs and curriculum at the University of Iowa College of Medicine, and he has also served in admissions and financial aid capacities at the Hahnemann Medical College and the University of Connecticut School of Medicine. A nationally known expert on medical school admissions, Mr. Taylor has held a number of leadership positions in national and regional medical student affairs organizations.

CONTRIBUTORS

Michael S. Katz, financial aid consultant for part six of this book, is the university director of student financial aid at the University of Medicine and Dentistry of New Jersey. He has been in the field of financial assistance, primarily in the health professions, for 25 years. Mr. Katz has served on numerous state, regional, and national education committees and has given presentations on financing a medical education. He is also a consultant to the U.S. Department of Health and Human Services.

Cynthia Lewis, Ph.D., author of chapters 13 and 15, received her doctorate in zoology from the University of Alberta in 1975, and held postdoctoral fellowships from the National Institute of Dental Research and Scripps Institution of Oceanography before becoming the preprofessional health adviser at San Diego State University (SDSU) for eleven years. She initiated and directed the SDSU Health Careers Opportunity grant for disadvantaged students from 1990–96, and is the founding prehealth adviser for the Collegiate Union for Health Related Education (CUHRE). Currently she is president of Lewis Associates Medical Strategies (www.lewisassoc.com), which provides personal premedical training and coaching to applicants pursuing a career in medicine.

Allen Maniker, M.D., author of chapter 17, is a board certified neurological surgeon and an assistant professor in the Division of Neurosurgery at the New Jersey Medical School in Newark, New Jersey. He received his M.D. from Wayne State University in 1986. He did an internship and one year of general surgery residency at New York's Beth Israel Medical Center and a residency and chief residency in neurological surgery at the New Jersey Medical School. He was a clinical fellow in neurotrauma at the Medical College of Virginia and a Clinical Fellow in peripheral nerve at the Louisiana State University in New Orleans and the University of Washington in Seattle. Dr. Maniker is director of neurotrauma and head of the New Jersey Peripheral Nerve Center at the New Jersey Medical School. He also holds an undergraduate degree from the Juilliard School in New York.

Elizabeth "Leah" Parker, who contributed to chapter 9, was affiliated with the University of California at Irvine College of Medicine from 1980 to 1997, serving as director of admissions for 12 years. During her tenure, she read and critiqued thousands of personal statement essays. Ms. Parker earned a master's degree in public administration from the California State University in Fullerton.

Chris Rosa, author of chapter 16, is director of the Office of Services for Students with Disabilities at Queens College, where he coordinates the provision of support services to more than 450 students with disabilities. A member of the Muscular Dystrophy Association's National Task Force on Public Awareness, Mr. Rosa has written several articles published in scholarly journals on the sociology of disability and is a recipient of the Muscular Dystrophy Association's National Personal Achievement Award. He is currently enrolled in a doctoral program in sociology at the City University of New York Graduate Center.

Rochelle Rothstein, M.D., received an honors degree in biology from Princeton University. An alumna of Kaplan's MCAT program, she received her M.D. from the University of California at San Diego. Dr. Rothstein is currently the vice president of Kaplan Medical, the division of Kaplan responsible for educational products for medical students and physicians. A recognized expert on the MCAT, medical school admissions, and U.S. medical licensure, Dr. Rothstein has lectured at universities and medical schools around the United States.

Charles Spooner, Jr., Ph.D., contributed to chapter 9. He has been involved in every aspect of medical school admissions, from initial recruitment to final selection and admission of students, for 27 years. Dr. Spooner is past national chairman of the Group on Student Affairs of the Association of American Medical Colleges, and has served several times on all the AAMC committees concerning admissions. He is currently a professor emeritus and associate dean emeritus of the University of California at San Diego School of Medicine.

A Special Note for International Students

Gaining admission to U.S. medical schools can be especially challenging for students who are not United States citizens. In recent years, less than one percent of first-year med school students were non-U.S. citizens. Most of these students attended college in the United States prior to applying to medical school.

If you are an international student interested in learning more about American medical and health care systems, or if you are considering attending medical school in the United States, Kaplan can help you explore your options. Here are some things you will want to consider if you are considering applying to attend med school in the United States.

> ## Oh, Canada
>
> Canadian readers interested in attending medical school in the United States should contact:
>
> Office of Public Affairs
> U.S. Embassy
> 490 Sussex Drive
> Ottawa, ON K1N 1G8
> Canada
> Tel: (613) 688-5391

- If English is not your first language, most medical schools will require you to take the computer or paper-and-pencil version of the TOEFL (Test of English as a Foreign Language) or provide some other evidence that you are proficient in English.

- Plan to take the MCAT; most U.S. medical schools require it.

- Begin the process of applying to medical schools at least eighteen months before the fall of the year you plan to start your studies. Most programs will only have September start dates.

- In addition, you will need to obtain an I-20 Certificate of Eligibility from the school you plan to attend if you intend to apply for an F-1 Student Visa to study in the United States.

- If you've already completed medical training outside the United States, get information about taking the United States Medical Licensing Exam (USMLE).

Kaplan International Programs

If you need more help with the complex process of medical school admissions, assistance preparing for the MCAT, USMLE, NCLEX or TOEFL, or help building your English language skills in general, you may be interested in Kaplan's programs for international students.

Kaplan International Programs were designed to help students and professionals from outside the United States meet their educational and career goals. At locations throughout the United States, international students take advantage of Kaplan's programs to help them improve their academic and conversational English skills, raise their scores on the TOEFL, MCAT, USMLE, and other standardized exams, and gain admission to the schools of their choice. Our staff and instructors give international students the individualized attention they need to succeed. Here is a brief description of some of Kaplan's programs for international students:

General Intensive English

Kaplan's General Intensive English classes are designed to help you improve your skills in all areas of English and to increase your fluency in spoken and written English. Classes are available for beginning to advanced students, and the average class size is 12 students.

English for TOEFL and University Preparation

This course provides you with the skills you need to improve your TOEFL score and succeed in an American university or graduate program. It includes advanced reading, writing, listening, grammar and conversational English, plus university admissions counseling. You will also receive training for the TOEFL using Kaplan's exclusive computer-based practice materials.

MCAT Test-Preparation Course

If you plan to enter a medical school in the United States, Kaplan can help you prepare for the MCAT. Kaplan also offers professional counseling and advice to help you gain a greater understanding of the American education system. We can help you with every step in the admissions process, from choosing the right medical school, to writing your application, to preparing for an interview.

Medical English Communication Review Course

This program is for international doctors and medical professionals. Lessons include mastering pronunciation, building your medical vocabulary, and developing presentation and legal writing skills. This program helps you develop the English skills you will need for the CSA exam, professional interviews, and interactions with patients.

Other Kaplan Programs

Since 1938, more than 3 million students have come to Kaplan to advance their studies, prepare for entry to American universities, and further their careers. In addition to the above programs, Kaplan offers courses to prepare for the SAT, GMAT, GRE, LSAT, DAT, USMLE, NCLEX, and other standardized exams at locations throughout the United States.

Applying to Kaplan International Programs

To get more information, or to apply for admission to any of Kaplan's programs for international students and professionals, contact us at:

Kaplan International Programs
888 Seventh Avenue
New York, NY 10106 USA
Telephone: (212) 492-5990 Fax: (212) 957-1654
E-mail: world@kaplan.com
Web: www.studyusa.kaplan.com

Kaplan is authorized under federal law to enroll nonimmigrant alien students.

Kaplan is authorized to issue Form IAP-66 needed for a J-1 (Exchange Visitor) visa.

Kaplan is accredited by ACCET (Accrediting Council for Continuing Education and Training).

Test names are registered trademarks of their respective owners.

PART ONE

Is Medical School for You?

CHAPTER 1

Making the Decision

Deciding to be a doctor is probably one of the most intimidating decisions you can make. As a premed student, you'll be working for at least two years without guarantee of a spot in medical school. It means publicly stating that you want something that in 1999 only 42 percent of those applying got—a position in medical school. After an arduous application process, that decision means committing to a labor-intensive course of study, including four years of medical school and three to twelve years of residency and fellowship.

Yet for all this, applications to med school are still quite high. There were 38,529 applicants for the class entering medical school in the fall of 1999. And while the number of candidates has actually decreased by about 6 percent over the last year, the number of medical school positions is a mere 16,200. That means that there are close to 2.5 times as many applicants as there are spots in medical schools. In this competitive environment, you need to prepare an application strategy carefully.

One important element of preparing your application campaign is articulating why you want to be a doctor; it's likely that you'll have to voice your desire in your personal statement, as well as in your interview. This also involves

> ### What's Up, Doc?
>
> Here are a handful of reasons medicine is a rewarding profession:
>
> - Patient rapport
> - Job responsibility
> - Lifetime learning
> - Great colleagues
> - Helping others
> - Job diversity
> - Financial satisfaction
> - Contact with people
> - Community respect
> - Science/research

demonstrating that you have glimpsed the reality of what it is to practice medicine, not the glamorized versions on *Chicago Hope* or *E.R.*

While some students have had a clear epiphany regarding their career goal that they can movingly relate, for many applicants, the decision to enter the medical field isn't as easily conveyed. Some find themselves daydreaming in organic chemistry class, still trying to decide two years into the prerequisites if this is the career for them. Complicating matters is the fact that many people want to be doctors for reasons that are not purely altruistic—for example, money, job security, or parental approval.

Are there legitimate reasons to decide to become a doctor? How can you figure out what's important to an admissions committee? How can you be honest about goals and aspirations that aren't particularly noble? It's important to address these questions as early as you can in the application process, and think through your own personal goals before you apply.

Why Go? Good Reasons . . .

There are a number of compelling reasons to become a doctor.

An Intimate Rapport

Being a physician gives you the most privileged listening post a human being can have. A doctor gets to hear the innermost issues of a patient, and is privileged to weave those hints and facts into a diagnosis and treatment.

Unique Responsibility

Doctors are at the top of the "medical food chain." At the hospital level, physicians work on a team with the nurses, therapists, and technicians who are taking care of a patient. The physician, however, has the voice that will carry the most weight. Physicians will be expected to make the difficult decisions: to decide when to stop life support, to declare that the slide under the microscope shows cancerous cells, even to carry the weight of prescribing a common antibiotic that can rarely cause lethal reactions. (This responsibility can also extend outside of the professional realm. On a plane or at a cocktail party, people will come up to you as a doctor and start telling you things about their skin you never wanted to know!)

Personal Tragedy

"I was 8 years old when my mother died of ovarian cancer. I remember dreaming of being a doctor then, thinking that maybe I could save her. I grew up without her guidance, but losing her sensitized me to the pain of others and played an important part in my decision to become a doctor."

—Univ. of Iowa College of Medicine student; adapted from Newsweek/Kaplan's *How to Choose a Career and Graduate School*

Special Authority

Many people pursue medicine because they want the knowledge of what to do in an emergency, and the ability to personally provide care for those in need. Some like the idea of being able to control things that were frightening or nebulous to them as children, while for others, the idea of being in a small town and being the one charged to take care of the whole town's health is appealing.

Other Reasons

In a recent poll, physicians reported other elements that lured them into the profession, among them:

- Continuing intellectual challenge
- Intelligent colleagues
- Joy of helping/taking care of people
- Respect of others in community
- Diversity of opportunities
- Opportunity to work with people
- Enjoyment of working with science or contributing to research
- Job autonomy and security
- Financial reward

As you think about why you are interested in medicine, make sure that you can articulate a goal such as those listed above. While financial reward and job security are indeed important, there are numerous other careers that provide these elements as well. What's important is that you can explain why medicine is your chosen profession.

Reasons to Reconsider

Many people experience the desire to be a doctor well before they are in a position to draw up any conscious list of goals—when they are still children. Though it may seem desirable to make a commitment early in life, it's important that you reconsider decisions you may have made as a child from an adult perspective. If you're applying to med school for any of the reasons listed below, examine your motivations before you take the plunge.

Parental Approval

Saying you want to be a doctor, even as a child, evokes pleased responses from adults. If you're someone who's always want-

Gotta Love It

A college senior we recently spoke to said that he wanted to be a doctor because it was the most difficult thing he could do. He worked hard to ace his MCAT, became volunteer coordinator of his fraternity, and selected his courses on the basis of how they'd look to an admissions committee. Sadly, a real desire to enter the field wasn't there, and admissions committees could tell: He hasn't yet gotten into med school.

ed to be a doctor, you might be able to remember how your goal was received early in your life. Making your career decision early isn't necessarily bad, as long as you've progressed beyond the approval-seeking stage. Until you've analyzed your commitment with an adult mind, you can't really argue successfully why you believe in it. You need to have a realistic sense of the profession, and of why you want to be a doctor, to convince a committee they should let you in.

The Longest Path

Another faulty reason is "the difficulty of the path." It's sometimes the case that high achievers pursue a career in medicine simply because it is so competitive, and involves such a lengthy, arduous path. Though stick-to-it-iveness and the discipline to accomplish a difficult goal are valuable assets in life and prized by medical school admissions officers, they alone are not enough. The alchemy of desire and motivation has to precede the chemistry of mixing the right MCAT scores, letters of recommendation, and extracurriculars. Real desire should be there.

Following in Mom or Dad's Footsteps

Many medical school applicants are children of physicians. Though having a parent who practices medicine may indeed give you a sense of the field, be aware that your folks went to medical school in a different era, and attending med school and starting to practice medicine have changed significantly in recent years. Some med school admissions officers estimate that children of physicians have a higher rate of attrition from medical school than the national average of one to two percent. It isn't that they can't do the work; it's that they sometimes discover they applied for the wrong reasons. If you are a child of a physician, give some extra thought to why you want to practice medicine in today's health care climate. This climate is characterized by the following:

Greater Competition

If your mother or father is in her or his forties or fifties, it's likely that she or he attended medical school around 25–30 years ago. At that time, the odds of getting into school were a bit better than 50 percent, as compared to less than 40 percent now. In addition, the pool of applicants was much smaller. The MCAT your parent took was a very different test: It carried far less weight than today's test does, and test takers did not usually prepare for it as carefully. Today, some test prep professionals estimate that almost 75 percent of the people who take the MCAT take a commercial test-prepara-

---

Changing Climate

The spread of HMOs and managed care is shaking the hierarchy of medical specializations and eroding physicians' incomes. Primary care physicians, who are much in demand by HMOs, are the gainers: since 1990 their incomes have jumped nearly 30 percent. As a result, more than half of all graduating medical students now enter programs in internal, family, or pediatric medicine.

—Adapted from Newsweek/Kaplan's *How to Choose a Career and Graduate School*

---

tion course. Finally, back around 1970, volunteering in a health-related situation wasn't included on the list of the AAMC's "Most Important Criteria" for admission. As of 1999, it is one of the big five.

Changing Medical Climate

Today's medical lingo is peppered with acronyms—HMO, DRGs, PPO, HIPC—that were not a part of medicine a generation ago. For that reason, don't assume that because you grew up with medicine you know what it's like. Today's private practice work is often signing papers in triplicate; in a public hospital, quadruplicate. Litigation and malpractice worries abound. It is not as easy to make a lot of money in the medical profession as it used to be. Look into these issues, so you can go into practice with your eyes wide open.

> ### Don't Do It for the Money
>
> "No amount of money is worth this amount of work. Don't get me wrong, there is money to be had, but the money is not worth it as a motivation. The most important advice is to get a life and keep it."
>
> —Medical student, University of California at Davis

What Med School Is Really Like

It's easy to nurture a fantasy of what med school will be like: Within days of your arrival, you'll be caring for patients, following eminent physicians, and, when you're done with a hard but reasonable day's work, you'll be leading a social life worthy of an upscale beer commercial.

Not surprisingly, few students report that their experience met their expectations. To many, med school is surprisingly reminiscent of high school, full of anxiety, pressure, and rigid scheduling.

Lingering Worries

After the exhilaration of being accepted and moving to a new place wears off, many students are left with the secret suspicion that everyone else in the orientation room had better scores and grades. The residual fear of "What if I never get accepted?" comes back in the form of "What if they find out I'm a fraud and I'm that one percent that never graduates?" No matter how often people tell you not to worry, some of that feeling remains.

Unbending Schedules

In college you could choose to skip class if you were burnt out. You probably had an hour or two of free time between class blocks. But the medical school format bears a stronger resemblance to high school. In a traditional curriculum, all 100-odd of your classmates stay in one room for a 50-minute class. When that class is over, the next professor/doctor puts her carousel of slides into the projector, and another 50-minute class on a different subject begins. Afternoon classes may be punctuated by labs. During the first year, two or three afternoons a week are typically anatomy lab, with dissection assignments that will often take you late into the wee hours of the morning to finish.

Delayed Gratification

Many students expect to jump right in and start taking care of patients. But the reality is that there's a whole world of knowledge you need before you're really able to care for people's medical needs. After years of dreaming about applying all your schooling, it's difficult to put that off for even longer.

Stress City

Part of the selection process for med school is designed to find out how much stress you've faced and how you've handled it. For that reason, you may get questions in an interview such as "What's the hardest thing you've ever had to do?" or "How do you handle stress?" Med school is admittedly stressful. The toughest part seems to be the quantity of material to be dealt with. All subjects are important, and there truly is more information than you could possibly learn. Someone else has always learned more than you about something, and particularly during the first year, there are always acronyms or diseases you've never heard of. Since most medical students are accustomed to being at the top of their classes, it's hard to get used to being one of the crowd, and perhaps no longer at the top.

Medical school administrations are well aware of student stress, and have programs in place to help students when they need it. The students who tend to do best are those who don't underestimate the difficulty of the work, who form study groups, and who make time for regular social events. Anticipating the stress is a good defense as well, as is believing that everyone else really is experiencing the same difficulties as you. And remember, even the person who graduates last in the class is called "doctor."

Decent Social Life

For many students, this is a pleasant surprise. Once most people adjust to med school, they find they have about as much social life as they had in college. It just has to be more carefully timed. Many mothers and fathers manage to care for their

---

The Hardest Years

"Before I entered residency, I thought med school was the four hardest years of my life. The amount of information you had to handle was overwhelming at times. Classes were very much like having a nine-to-five job, and then you had to go home and memorize all the information in the evening."

—M.D., University of North Carolina, Chapel Hill, 1994

As for Residents...

Despite efforts to reform the system, young doctors doing their residencies still work inhumanly long days. "I've operated when I've been up for 24 hours," says Jana Kaplan, a third-year Ob-Gyn resident in Baltimore County, MD, who puts in 100-hour weeks even though she is pregnant.

—Adapted from Newsweek/Kaplan's *How to Choose a Career and Graduate School*

families while doing well in medical school; it's just a matter of prioritizing and scheduling.

Life in medical school revolves around the testing schedule. Some schools have all tests on one day three or four times a semester. This means that the weekend after a test day is totally free, and you can go camping, party, or spend time with your family. Other schools will have tests throughout the year; you'll learn to schedule weekend fun that includes a few hours away from everyone to study for your biochemistry quiz the following Monday.

Peers and Colleagues

For some people, medical school is the first social group in which everyone wants to do basically the same things, and everyone has had to prepare academically in basically the same way. You'll find many things in common with everyone in your class. There's a flip side, though: While medical schools aim for diversity, your classmates may be a surprisingly homogeneous group. One hundred or so people is usually large enough for you to find a core group you like, but it may make for a smaller circle of friends than you're used to.

Friends

The changes most medical students notice in their social lives are:

- Having to say "no" to nonmed school friends who want to go out
- Losing touch with some more peripheral friends from college and other cities
- Becoming aware that their day-to-day vocabulary has become quite different from that of their nonmedical friends
- Giving in to the urge to "talk shop" while socializing

Married Life

It's no secret that med school can stress a relationship, whether one or both individuals are attending. However, plenty of couples happily survive those four years. Most medical schools, especially those affiliated with larger universities, have activities for students' spouses or partners. Married medical students are making up more of each med class. Since students begin medical school, on the average, at age 22 and graduate at 26, lots of students partner up during their medical school years. Typically, between 5–15 percent of an entering class will be married, and 40–70 percent of a graduating class will be married. Chances are if you're married or in a committed relationship, you'll be able to find other couples with similar interests from within your own class.

The bottom line is that while med school is different from what you might have expected, and certainly stressful for most people, it's not prison. Many enjoy their experience, make lasting friendships, and are able to nurture the relationships that matter to them.

The Qualities Schools Are Looking For

One important consideration in your decision to become a doctor is whether you are the kind of person who is well suited to a medical career. In other words, you have to ask yourself if you will make a good doctor. This can be a difficult question to answer since there is no one model to which you can compare yourself. The reason for this is obvious: Medicine is many different careers and many different kinds of people will do well in some aspect of medicine. For example, it takes a different set of skills to be a transplant surgeon than it does to be a psychiatrist. Medical schools differ widely in the kind of students they seek. Furthermore, each medical school will attempt to enroll a wide variety of students in the belief that this diversity will enrich the educational experience of all students.

While there is no one model for the ideal medical student and physician, there are a number of qualities that most medical schools find desirable in their applicants. Ask yourself how you rate in each characteristic.

Cognitive Ability

Native intelligence is essential. It takes intellectual firepower to learn and understand the body of knowledge required to be a doctor. This is why medical schools place such emphasis on your academic record.

Critical Thinking

Knowledge by itself is not enough. Doctors must be able to think critically, to synthesize information, and to solve problems. They must be able to find the answers to puzzles and to tease out a diagnosis from a set of often unclear, ambiguous, or contradictory facts or symptoms. This ability is one aspect of what has been called the art of medicine. The problem-solving nature of much of the MCAT is an indicator of the emphasis that medical schools place on this quality.

Curiosity

You need to have a sincere desire to investigate and to learn. Much of the knowledge you gain in medical school will be out of date within a few years of your graduation. You must have the desire to keep learning new things, to be a life-long learner. Do you have a sense of wonder about how the body works? About what causes disease? About how things work? Do you follow through to find answers to questions like these?

Lifelong Learning

"We are in the midst of the most dramatic medical advances in history, and there will be much more to come. To be a doctor or medical researcher, be prepared to be a lifelong learner."

—Dr. William A. Peck, Washington University School of Medicine

Commitment

The rewards of being a doctor are many, but in order to reap those rewards you must be committed to working harder than most people. The hours are long and so is the period of training. In fact, your medical education never ends. You need to be dedicated to spending your entire career keeping up, learning new things, staying on top. As a doctor, you will be given the opportunity to help your patients in their most trying times, but this means that they will ask much of you. They will want you to be there when they need you and to be willing to do what it takes to help them recover from illness. You must really want to be a doctor and be willing to make the sacrifices needed to become an excellent one. The drive should come from inside. You should feel emotionally impelled to be a doctor.

Compassion

A compassionate person is one who is conscious of others' distress and who has a sincere desire to alleviate that distress. Most people considering careers in medicine say that they want to help people. This is the heart of medicine. There is no better way to show compassion than by dedicating yourself to helping others regain or maintain their health. Ask yourself what you have done to demonstrate that you are compassionate. Medical schools will want to see some evidence that you possess this quality.

Communication Skills

A doctor must be able to communicate well. One of the most frequently heard complaints voiced by patients is that their doctors won't listen to them, or conversely, that their doctors won't talk to them. Highly developed communication skills are essential. Work at developing your communication skills by actively participating in out-of-class activities that allow you to interact with others and that require you to be an effective communicator.

Cooperation

Cooperation means acting or working with others; in other words, teamwork. Doctors must be able to work closely and cooperatively with colleagues from many specialties. Moreover, doctors do not work alone. Health care today involves a variety of professionals: nurses; therapists; technicians; and others. The effective doctor is one who recognizes the contribution each person can make to the care of the patient and who can participate with them as a member of the health care team. Ask yourself how well you work with others. Do you insist on "doing it yourself" or are you willing to involve others?

Cultural Awareness

We live in a multicultural society. As a doctor you will treat patients from many cultures vastly different from your own. Their customs, beliefs, social forms, and truths may diverge greatly from the ones you were taught. You will need to be aware of and sensitive to those differences in order to effectively communicate with and help those patients. This goes beyond tolerance of differences; you will need to try to understand those differences.

Character

Physicians are given a special place in society. Medicine is consistently rated as one of the most highly regarded professions in America. Doctors are granted access to their patients' most private secrets and are given powers over their patients few others are privileged to possess. With these privileges comes a high level of responsibility. We demand much of our doctors. As a physician you will be held to an exceptionally high standard of moral excellence and firmness. Your character must be above reproach, your values unquestioned.

How Hard Is It to Get In?

Getting into medical school will be one of your most difficult challenges in seeking a career in medicine. While the number of applicants to medical school has been dropping a little in recent years, competition remains sharp. In 1999 there were 2.4 applicants for every place available in allopathic medical schools in the United States. To put it another way, only 42.1 percent of applicants were admitted in 1999. It is reasonable to assume that many of the applicants who were not admitted were good candidates who would have made good doctors. Obviously you will need dedication and careful planning to be successful in this competitive situation.

Your Premed Adviser

If you're having doubts about whether med school is for you, or wondering about your chances of getting in, the best thing to do is to talk to your premed adviser. He or she can help you decide if you should apply to medical school, can help assess your chances of getting in, and can guide you to the right schools, both in terms of the best curriculum for your interests and the most likely schools that will accept you. Your premed adviser will have specific data about med school requirements, how students from your school fared in the admissions process, and where students with similar academic backgrounds and MCAT scores were accepted.

Going It Alone

Naturally, you can choose to apply to medical school without the help of the premed office. But medical schools are usually familiar with the procedures of different undergrad institutions. If they know you had access to a premed office, they will almost certainly wonder why you chose to bypass it.

At many undergraduate institutions, the premed office handles the letters of recommendation. In some cases, they simply relay the letters to the medical schools. In other cases, the premed adviser or committee writes a letter to the admissions offices on your behalf. This letter can take the form of a "composite letter" which excerpts your recommendations, or it may simply be a cover letter that accompanies the recommendations. Either way, it is imperative that you get to know the people who are going to be writing letters on your behalf. In most such cases, the adviser(s) will require a certain number of meetings with their advisees. Take these meetings very seriously.

With the number of applications to medical school at an all-time high, premed advisers are a harried bunch these days. It's possible that if you're not a particularly strong candidate, you may find your adviser less than enthusiastic about your applying to medical school. He or she may have legitimate concerns about your competitiveness and may try to dissuade you from applying. Then it's up to you. You may have to go it alone without the full support of your school's premed office. Be realistic. If everyone agrees your chances are slim, have a backup plan just in case you're not admitted.

If you do not know if there is an advisor at your school you may be able to find out through The National Association of Advisors to the Health Professions (NAAHP). The NAAHP publishes the names of advisors on undergraduate college campuses on its web site. It also has a list of advisors who have agreed to work with applicants whose college does not have an advisor. Look at the NAAHP web site, www.naahp.org to find these lists.

The Bottom Line

Before you apply, and before you start diving into the heavy premed prerequisites, take some time to seriously evaluate why you want to go to med school, if you'd consider alternative careers in health care, and what you'll do if you don't get in. If nothing else, doing so will give you a leg up on the admissions process, and a chance to express your goals before you're asked to do so in a personal statement or interview.

The next step in your journey is to plan out your undergraduate years, including what classes you need to take, and which extracurricular activities you should consider.

PART TWO

Planning for Medical School

CHAPTER 2

Planning Your Undergraduate Curriculum

Success requires a good plan, hard work, and a little luck. This is particularly true of the pursuit of a medical career. While there is little we can do about the last two parts of the equation, we can help you develop your plan to apply successfully to medical school.

All plans have a beginning. To be a successful medical school applicant, you need to treat your quest for admission as a strategic campaign. You have to put your best foot forward—first on paper, then in person. The more you understand about the application process, and the more time and care you dedicate to approaching the process (both in research and preparation), the better your chances are of gaining admission to medical school.

Undergraduate Basics

The first step in planning for a medical education is to plan your undergraduate education. Medical schools are looking for well-rounded, broadly educated students. That said, there are still many decisions that you will need to make.

Picking the "Right" Undergraduate College

Premed students and their parents are often concerned with going to the "right" undergraduate school, meaning that undergraduate school that will give the student the greatest chance of getting into medical school. As much as we hate to admit it, there is some validity to this attitude, given that most medical school admission committees do consider the undergraduate institution attended when reviewing an applicant's academic history. However, a particular medical school's admissions committee's opinion of an undergraduate institution shouldn't be the litmus test for whether you should attend that college. First, it's highly unlikely that a medical school will give you its rankings of undergraduate schools. Second, it would be difficult to get most, much less all, medical schools to agree as to the quality of education at any given undergraduate institution. Third, the four or more years you will spend getting your undergraduate education are more that just a pit stop on your way to medical school. College should be a time of exploration, development, and maturation from an emotional, spiritual, physical, and intellectual perspective. Finally, as hard as this is to believe, you may ultimately decide you want to do something else with your life than become a physician.

Considering all this, a better way to approach the issue of where to attend undergraduate school is to compile of list of schools you believe will enable you to do your best work. Ask yourself the following questions:

- Do you do better work on a quarter system or a semester system? Do you hit the ground running at the introduction to a new subject matter but suffer from a short attention span, or do you take a while to warm up but come on strong at the end?
- Would you do better in a small class size environment (fewer than 100) in which you would be more likely to get individual attention, or do you prefer the stimulation, as well as the anonymity, of a large class size (greater than 500)?
- Would you like to be within driving distance of home and therefore able to take advantage of an occasional home-cooked meal and laundry service, or when you leave the nest do you need to get as far away as possible?

Two-Year versus Four-Year Colleges

Many successful applicants complete part of their undergraduate education at a two-year community college. The reasons for doing so include an initial inability to gain admission to a four-year institution, financial considerations, course selection and availability, and issues of convenience. While you certainly can take some courses at a two-year school, whenever possible, complete your prerequisite science courses at a four-year institution. Many admissions committees look to your performance in undergraduate science courses as being a good predictor of your potential to negotiate the preclinical medical school curriculum. Therefore, you should strive to perform well in the most academically challenging environment available to you. Typically, although not always, this means completing prerequisite coursework at a four-year college or university.

An additional factor for consideration is that many admissions committees do not consider grades earned from community colleges when evaluating your composite GPA. If you have taken all of your science courses at a community college and you apply to a medical school that does not consider community college grades, you could find yourself without a science GPA for the purposes of that particular medical school.

These are just some of the many issues you might consider when deciding whether or not a particular college or university is right for you. Remember, it doesn't do you or anyone else any good for you to go to the "right" school if you crash and burn because it wasn't the school that was "right" for you.

Once you've made your list of schools you believe would enable you to get the most out of your undergraduate experience, then, and only then, should you consider how the institution rates with medical schools. You can do this by inquiring of the premed office what percentage of premed applicants were accepted over the past five years. Compare that number to the percentage accepted within the state as well as across the country (both of which are available in the *Medical School Admission Requirements*, also known as the MSAR—more on this valuable resource in chapter 4). Ideally, the school you attend should have acceptance rates equal to or higher than both the state and national averages. For more information, consider turning to your high school guidance counselor, science instructors, family physician, and commercial publications such as Newsweek/Kaplan's *How to Get Into College*.

> ### Straight from the Source
>
> For a complete listing of accredited schools, get the current year's directory of *Medical School Admission Requirements (MSAR)* by contacting:
>
> Association of American Medical Colleges
> Attn: Publication Orders
> 2450 N Street, N.W.
> Washington, DC 20037
> (202) 828-0416
> www.aamc.org
>
> Cost $25.00 plus $6.00 shipping

Choosing an Undergraduate Major

As we've already said, admissions committees look for well-rounded, broadly educated applicants. Successful candidates demonstrate a high level of scholastic achievement and intellectual curiosity, as well as an aptitude for the sciences.

As a rule, admissions committees do not give "credit" for a candidate's undergraduate major. Therefore, aside from doing well in the required premedical courses, it is important for you to choose a major of your liking. This is important for two reasons: First, your overall academic record will probably be stronger if you take classes you enjoy; and second, if you choose not to go to medical school, you will have a major that will aid you in either gaining employment or in applying to graduate school.

> ### Do What You Like
>
> Don't choose a major because you think it will get you accepted to med school. Choose to major in something you're really interested in studying. You'll probably get better grades if you study what interests you most.

In its listing of information regarding the majors of successful medical school applicants, the MSAR notes that nearly 38 percent were bio majors; science majors in general comprised about 65 percent of those accepted to med schools in 1999. This might lead you to believe that medical schools prefer science majors. This is not necessarily true: Note that the acceptance rates of certain humanities majors were equal to or greater than those of science majors. For instance, last year, approximately 40 percent of the biology majors who applied were accepted, while approximately 50 percent of the history and philosophy majors were accepted.

Of course, this doesn't mean that medical schools prefer *nonscience* majors. What these statistics indicate is that if you're a nonscience major, you're not at a disadvantage. The more important basis for admission to med school is your undergraduate transcript, no matter what your major is. If you're not a science major, your work in both science and nonscience courses will be evaluated. However, with fewer courses on which to judge your science ability, your grades in the core science courses will take on greater importance.

On the other hand, a science major who has taken the minimum of nonscience courses may in fact be at some disadvantage: Medicine is a people profession, and many admissions committees look for applicants with demonstrated interests in the world around them, which may be illustrated in part by a broad selection of courses.

Basic Course Requirements

The faculty at each medical school is responsible for establishing courses required for admission. In some cases, required courses reflect courses needed for licensure as a physician in the state in which the medical school is located; in other cases, prerequisites reflect institutional requirements.

In general, requirements include one year of biology, one year of physics, one year of general chemistry, and one year of organic chemistry, as well as each subject's related lab work. Additionally, many medical schools also require math and English. The best sources for specific information on prerequisites are the MSAR, which lists requirements for all accredited allopathic medical schools, and the *College Information Booklet*, which has similar information on all of the country's osteopathic medical schools.

Selecting Your Prerequisite Courses

When enrolling in your required premed courses, you will almost always have a choice of two different course sequences to take: courses for students majoring in that particular discipline, and courses for everyone else. For example, when you register to take the one-year general physics requirement, you will have the option of taking a one-year general physics sequence for physics majors, or a one-year general physics sequence for nonmajors. If you happen to be a physics major, the decision is easy—you take the sequence designed for physics majors. However, what if you're not a physics major? Which sequence should you take?

In general, medical school admissions committees state that when two course sequences are available, you should take the more academically challenging of the two. That said, there are still some practical realities of life that you might want to consider. First, the reason why many college subjects are divided into two distinct tracts for majors or nonmajors is because the subject matter is difficult. Courses designed for students majoring in that discipline are filled with students who live, eat, and breathe the stuff, and are therefore presumably good at it. The competition will be stiff. If you think you can do well, go for it. But if you think you will have to work very hard to perform in the middle of the class, it is probably wiser to take the sequence for the nonmajors.

This brings us to the second practical reality of life: It is unlikely that the medical school admissions committee reviewing your application will be fully versed as to the course sequences offered by your undergraduate institution, or that they will actually reward you for having chosen to take the harder sequence for each of your premed requirements. What is more likely to be true is that your application will be considered based upon your academic performance without regard for whether or not you took the more difficult sequence.

Does that mean you should endeavor to "pad" your GPA by taking the easiest courses available? No. Not only will this type of behavior inevitably catch up with you, but it is not a personality trait that admissions committees, or patients, are looking for in future physicians. But it does mean you should use your head. Challenge yourself, yes. Push yourself to develop your potential, yes. But don't put yourself in a position where you have no hope of succeeding academically no matter how hard you work.

A related issue concerns choice of instructors. It may be that the same class, taught by different instructors, is offered on different days or times. If you have a choice, by all means find out all you can about each instructor and his or her teaching style. You can do this by reading the course evaluations that are usually on file with the course department or student services, or by talking to upper classmen or your premed advisor. Once you have done your investigation, pick the instructor who is best for you and your learning style.

Scheduling of Prerequisite Courses

Unless you are in a structured postbaccalaureate program, you should endeavor to pace the completion of your prerequisite courses over your four undergraduate years.

Freshman Year

Typically, applicants complete the one-year general chemistry requirement during their freshman year. Other prerequisites typically taken during the freshman year include lower division biology (one semester), math (one semester), English (one semester) and other lower-division courses required for your major. Any associated laboratory courses are generally completed concurrently with the lecture portion of the course.

Sophomore Year

The sophomore year typically includes completion of the one-year organic chemistry requirement, lower-division biology (one semester), and other lower-division courses required for your major.

Junior Year

Med school applicants often complete the one-year physics requirement during the junior year, along with electives and any upper-division courses required for your major.

Senior Year

By this time, you should have completed all the prerequisites for medical school. Most students reserve the senior year for finishing up any requirements of their major, and for electives.

Waiving Requirements

Many applicants want to know whether requirements can be waived. Requirements cannot be waived if they are licensure requirements. However, institutional requirements may be waived depending on the institutional policy. Your best bet is to complete the prerequisite courses of those medical schools to which you plan to apply. If you are unable to complete a requirement, check with each relevant institution regarding their waiver policy.

AP Credit

Many applicants receive high school AP credit for lower-division science courses. AP credits can often satisfy prerequisite requirements. However, because this is an institutional decision, contact each school you're applying to regarding its policy.

Study Abroad

Many applicants have the opportunity at some time during their undergraduate careers to take advantage of opportunities to study abroad. If you are lucky enough to do so, congratulations: The chance to live, work, and play in a different culture will be one of the great experiences of your life. Because you will undoubtedly want to take advantage of travel and social opportunities while you are abroad, it is probably advisable that you do not overload your academic schedule. To this end, you should save any outstanding prerequisite courses until you return to your home undergraduate campus. You may also want to consider taking your courses pass-fail, particularly if you are studying in a country where the language spoken is not your native tongue.

Another important consideration is that you will most likely be applying to medical schools during your senior year. Since all medical schools require personal interviews, if you are engaged in study abroad during your application year, you may be required to return to the United States for interviews. Make sure that you (and your budget) allow for this possibility.

Undergraduate Degree

Most medical schools do not require a college degree. Rather, the typical requirement is that applicants have a minimum of three years of full-time undergraduate work at an accredited college or university. That said, the majority of successful applicants do hold a baccalaureate degree. Just what degree you are awarded is not important, since there is no distinction made between a bachelor of science and a bachelor of arts degree.

Postbaccalaureate Programs

Postbaccalaureate programs are academic programs specifically designed to help applicants improve their chances of gaining admission to medical school. While there are several types of postbac programs (discussed in chapters 12 and 13), one type is for students who decide to apply to medical school after graduation from college, and need to fulfill prerequisite course requirements, or wish to retake courses to improve their performance.

If you're considering entering a postbaccalaureate program, bear in mind that postbaccalaureate work is automatically averaged in with the undergraduate GPA on the American Medical College Application Service (AMCAS) application. The extent to which the postbac work is ultimately considered depends on the degree to which individual admissions committees consider it relevant to the evaluation process.

CHAPTER 3

Extracurricular Activities

Your undergraduate years should be a grand adventure, a time of tremendous growth and endless possibilities. They are a time to discover who you are, what you value, and how you fit into the larger world. They are a time of transition. In order to get as much as possible out of your college years, it is important that you do something other than study.

Medical school admissions committees select applicants who have demonstrated intelligence, maturity, integrity, and a dedication to the ideal of service to society. Of these qualities, your intelligence is the easiest to measure objectively. Assessment of the other three gets a little trickier, and a lot more subjective. Nonetheless, admissions committees have developed methods for doing so.

One way of assessing your nonacademic qualities is to look at how you have lived your life prior to completing your medical school application. To this end, many committees will ask you to submit a list of the extracurricular activities with which you have been involved. While not all admissions committees consider extracurricular activities in the application process, those that do consider the nature and depth of the extracurricular activities you have undertaken to be a significant factor in your admissibility to medical school.

Clinical Experience

Of all the activities you could be involved in, the one that is most likely to be considered essential by a medical school admissions committee is clinical experience. After all, you are applying to medical school, not business, law, or graduate school. It is not unreasonable for the committee to want to see some evidence of the fact that you have given thought to what you're getting into. The standard answer applicants give when asked why they want a career in medicine is, "I want to help people." While there is nothing wrong with that answer (one sure way to be eliminated from the competition is to say "I don't like helping people"), clearly you can help people and have a lot more "fun" as a cruise director than as a physician. Sick people don't feel well; they get cranky and they may forget to say "thank you." Admissions committees want proof that you have some sense of what you'll be getting in to.

What's the Best Experience?

The quintessential clinical experience an applicant can have is to work in an emergency room. Emergency rooms are plentiful and they're always looking for a few good volunteers. That said, the experience is seldom a good use of your time. The reason for this is that E.R.'s tend to be busy places. You don't know anything about emergency medicine. Therefore, what you'll most likely end up doing is running errands for someone. Not the best use of your time, given that the goal is for you to gain insight into the role that a physician plays in the health care delivery system.

Your time would be much better spent if you volunteered for a chronic care activity. By this we mean working with people who have a chronic illness or disability. Because these patients have long-term conditions, volunteers get put to real use as support individuals within the health care team. Additionally, you are likely to work with the same patient and their families for weeks, if not months, at a time. This can give you the opportunity to experience health care over time from multiple perspectives—that of the patient, his family, the physician, and other members of the health care delivery team.

Try the Hospital

"I recommend doing hospital volunteer work. It gives you the chance to find out if you like the work environment, being around sick people. And, best of all, it's fun. You'd be surprised how few prospective medical students list volunteer-work experience."

—Soni J. Anderson, University of Alabama School of Medicine, adapted from Newsweek/Kaplan's *How to Choose a Career and Graduate School*

How to Find It

The best way to find such an experience is to call those organizations in your community that work with the chronically ill or disabled. Such organizations may involve conditions such as multiple sclerosis, cystic fibrosis, mental retardation, battered women and children, spinal cord injuries, drug addicted babies, AIDS patients, and so on. Pick an organization of interest to you and go for it. Remember that you may be asked to make a commitment of up to one year, but in return you will be made a real member of the team.

Research Experience

In general, the only time research experience is an absolute must is if you are planning to apply to M.D./Ph.D. programs, or are representing yourself as someone who is interested in an academic or research career. If this is the case, then again it is important that you have documented experience that validates your interest and potential in the career field.

But that doesn't mean that applicants planning a pure clinical career wouldn't benefit from a research background. As a future physician, your job will involve research, either as you seek to determine your patients' medical conditions, or through the process of continuing education, in which you study other individuals' research efforts.

Most applicants obtain their research experience during the course of their undergraduate studies. There are three paths by which students usually obtain their first research experience. The first involves taking a class for academic credit that is designed to allow the student to work one-on-one with a faculty member on an independent research project. The second path involves applying and being accepted to participate in a sponsored summer research program. The final path entails volunteering in a laboratory and working your way up to a position of greater responsibility. This final option is the one most frequently utilized by students with no prior lab experience.

> ### Stand Out
>
> "Med school is so competitive that you have to find some way to distinguish yourself. I was an English major, had a musical background, and worked as an undergraduate, and I think these are all things that helped me stand out to some degree. Admissions people don't talk about applicants as 'the person with a 4.0 and great MCAT scores.' Virtually every applicant is at the top of his or her class, has great letters of recommendation, and was in an honors society. Admissions people remember the applicant who worked with handicapped children, started a soup kitchen, or had an art exhibit."
>
> —M.D., Jefferson Medical College, 1994

Teaching Experience

A third category of extracurricular activity common to many successful applicants is teaching. One of the most important roles that a physician plays is that of a teacher as she imparts information to her patients; teaching patients enables them to play a more active role in their own health care.

The diversity of teaching experiences of medical school applicants during their undergraduate years is very broad. Such experience might include teaching bible study in your place of worship, teaching swimming or a musical instrument to children, or becoming a teaching assistant in a lower-division class in which you did exceptionally well. Teaching can encompass just about anything you enjoy doing. All you need to do is share it with others in a structured, organized manner.

Employment

In today's economy, many undergraduate students need to work throughout their college years in order to stay in school. Many admissions committees recognize that the time you work necessarily means that you have less time for your studies and other forms of extracurricular activities. These committees understand that maintaining academic performance while holding down a job is hard work. If an applicant has been able to do both well, it is an indication that he will be able to maintain his academic performance upon entering medical school, when work demands are significantly decreased or eliminated, but academic pressures increase.

Other Activities

These are but a few of the types of activities that may be considered noteworthy by medical school admissions committees. Other activities may include participation in campus or community governance, membership on a varsity sports team, excellence in the arts, or the commitment of a significant amount of time to a socially meaningful activity such as the Peace Corp or AmeriCorp. Again, while not all med school admissions committees consider extracurricular activities a part of the evaluation process, many do. One warning, though: Under no circumstances should you expect that heavy participation in extracurricular activities will forgive a poor academic record. Your first priority must be to demonstrate academic excellence. Don't expect great understanding from committee members if your grades suffer as a result of participation in nonacademic activities. The committee's reaction is likely to be that you showed poor judgment in setting your priorities.

PART THREE

Selecting
a Program

CHAPTER 4

Your Basic Choices

Choosing the medical schools to which you will apply is a major decision. It's important that you take the time to research medical schools in which you're interested, so you'll be in a better position to match their criteria with yours. After reviewing this chapter, you'll be prepared to start drafting your list of schools.

The Basics

Unfortunately, many applicants know very little, if anything, about the medical schools to which they apply. They enter the application process blindly, and base their decisions on "common knowledge" or "school reputation." This is a naive way of planning a future. Before plunging into the actual logistics of the application process, you need to review some of the main criteria for selecting schools.

MSAR: Your Premed Bible

There are currently 122 accredited medical schools in the United States, three in Puerto Rico, and 16 in Canada. *Medical School Admission Requirements,* which is published every April and is affectionately called the "MSAR," provides comprehensive information on all of these schools. When it comes to med school admissions, "doing it by the book" refers to the MSAR. The information in this book comes from the horses' mouths—the schools themselves. It isn't filled with second-hand accounts or student opinions. It's the official stuff.

The first part of the MSAR includes over 100 pages relating to the admissions process. The second part includes profiles of all the Liaison Committee on Medical Education (LCME)–accredited schools in the

United States and Canada. It's worth the $25 you'll need to purchase your own copy, since the information in there can help you decide where to apply. Every school profiled in the MSAR contains the following entries:

- General information
- Curriculum
- Requirements
- Selection factors
- Early decision program
- Tuition
- Financial aid
- Application and acceptance policies
- Information on previous year's class

In chapter 5, we'll tell you how to make the most of this excellent resource.

Narrowing Down Your List

At some point, you're going to have to bite the bullet and narrow down your list of schools. While there is no magical number of schools to apply to, the average is now around 12 or 13 schools. (California applicants average closer to 25 schools.) Naturally, if you're going to apply to lots of very competitive schools, you may need to construct a more extensive list. Work with your premed advisor to select schools that make sense for you. Check to see where students from your college with your GPA and MCAT scores have been accepted. Also, inquire whether your school has a historical feeder relationship with a particular medical school.

While you're agonizing over which schools to keep on your list, consider the following issues:

- Competitiveness
- Cost
- Accreditation
- Curriculum
- Teaching hospitals
- Location
- Affiliation with undergraduate institutions
- Student body
- Public versus private schools

Competitiveness

As we mentioned in the introduction to this section, competition to get into medical school is very intense. You need to be realistic about your admission chances. There are many qualified applicants who won't be accepted. Don't take anything for granted; apply to schools of varying degrees of competitiveness.

The entire notion of ranking schools is, of course, a highly subjective and controversial exercise. However, rankings can provide an idea of how competitive it is to gain admission into a school. For instance, so-called Top Ten medical schools (e.g., UCSF, Hopkins, Harvard, Stanford, etcetera) are very competitive. For a somewhat more objective method of evaluating a particular school's competitiveness, check your MSAR.

> ## Don't Limit Yourself
>
> Don't skimp on the number of applications you make. Yes, it's expensive, but this is an important step. It pays to give yourself as much choice as possible.

It's helpful to view schools in categories: highly competitive schools; middle-tiered schools; and finally the backup or "safety" school. (These days, however, there really is no such thing as a safety school.) You should not take the risk of applying only to the most competitive schools—the outcome may be rejection from all of them.

By the way, don't get too hung up about a school's "reputation." All LCME-accredited schools provide a solid medical education and no matter where you go, you get the magical M.D. after your name.

Cost

You may have already taken out loans to pay your undergraduate education, or have mortgages or high rents to pay. Tuition to medical school will only add to your financial burden. Of the 122 LCME-accredited medical schools in the United States, 52 are private institutions and the rest are state sponsored. The difference in cost between attending a state and a private medical school can be striking. For example, consider the tuition at a state institution such as the University of Nevada Reno Medical School. In 1999–2000, tuition for a resident was $7,782, as opposed to $22,808 for a nonresident. While the cost for a nonresident is by no means pocket change, compare this to a private institution such as Georgetown Medical School. The tuition at Georgetown ran $29,940 for 1999–2000.

Remember, we're comparing only tuition. This doesn't figure in the cost of living (room, board, entertainment, etcetera). It is safe to say that the cost of living in Reno, Nevada, is significantly lower than in Washington, D.C. If you were a resident of Nevada, you'd be talking about a difference of at least $20,000; that's $80,000 in four years.

The solution seems all too obvious, right? Everyone should attend state schools! The problem: limited slots and strict residency requirements. State schools often strongly favor those applicants who are state residents (i.e., those who are already paying taxes to support the existence of the school). Unfortunately, residency requirements differ from state to state, so there is no one set way of establishing residency. Nonetheless, when considering the economics of going to medical school, state residency may become

Pros and Cons of the Military Option

"I applied for the Health Professions Scholarship Program with the Army. They pick up just about every cost that you can imagine, and give you a living stipend. In return, I had to go through officer basic training and rotations with the Army. The military is interested in keeping you happy, and you get to choose what sort of rotations you do. I have no regrets about following this path. If it wasn't for the financial support of the military, I'd probably be changing tires somewhere."

—M.D., Jefferson Medical College

"One problem with the military route is that we had very little real-world exposure. In the military, you tell someone to take medicine, it's an order. People are more likely to follow rules. It's different in the civilian world. We were taught how to deal with war, famine, and exodus. It's intimidating that at some point I will have to deal with the HMO world."

—M.D., Uniformed Services University of Health Sciences

a vital issue. It is important that you decide which state schools are feasible for you, and that you clear up any misconceptions concerning residency requirements well before you apply.

Accreditation

It is essential that the medical school you attend meets the standards established by the Liaison Committee on Medical Education (LCME), the body that is responsible for accrediting M.D.-granting programs in the United States. The LCME is made up of representatives appointed by the AAMC, the Council on Medical Education of the American Medical Association, the Committee on Accreditation of Canadian Medical Schools, as well as representatives of the general public.

LCME standards state that a medical school's curriculum must be designed to provide a general professional education, recognizing that this alone is insufficient to prepare a graduate for independent, unsupervised medical practice. The LCME requires schools to have a program that provides a minimum of 130 weeks of instruction, usually over at least four years, and that allows students to:

- Learn the fundamental principles of medicine

- Acquire the skills of clinical judgment based on evidence and experience

- Develop an ability to use principles and skills wisely in solving problems of health and disease

- Acquire an understanding of the scientific concepts underlying medicine

- Be introduced to current advances in the basic sciences, including therapy and technology, changes in the understanding of disease, and the effect of social needs and demands on medical care

The LCME goes on to specify a number of basic science and clinical areas that each medical school's curriculum must cover but it does not specify exactly how that curriculum must be organized. As a result, medical schools differ widely on how they present their educational programs.

Curriculum

Medical school alone will not prepare you to practice as a physician. What it will do is give you the basic training that you need to continue into residency training (graduate medical education) in the specialty that best suits your talents and interests. Only after you have completed residency training and have met other licensure requirements are you ready to enter medical practice on your own.

Because medical school lays the foundation for the rest of your medical career, the curriculum of the medical school you attend is one of the most important criteria in selecting schools to which you will apply.

For most of the twentieth century, medical school has been divided into two phases: preclinical (basic sciences) and clinical. Up until recently, students were exposed to a two-year intensive dose of the basic sciences before having any meaningful patient contact. The preclinical (also referred to as basic science) years were followed by two years of patient contact composed of clerkships and electives. The distinction between preclinical and clinical years has blurred somewhat in recent years as medical schools introduce students to earlier patient contact, often during the first year of the curriculum. Here are some of the ways in which medical school curricula differ today:

- Length
- Organization of the preclinical years
- Use of problem-based learning
- Organization of the clinical years
- Earliest patient contact
- Primary care focus
- Innovative educational methods and new technologies
- Student evaluation
- USMLE policies
- Special programs and opportunities

Length

The LCME requirement that schools offer a curriculum of at least 130 weeks of instruction has resulted in a standard, four-year program at nearly all medical schools. A few schools offer the opportunity for at least some students to take additional time (usually five years) to complete the program. Programs of fewer than four-years are relatively rare.

Organization of the Preclinical Years

Until relatively recently, the preclinical years of the medical curriculum were referred to as the basic science years. Students took traditional courses in disciplines such as anatomy, biochemistry, physiology, microbiology and immunology, pathology, pharmacology and therapeutics, and preventive medicine.

Instruction consisted of long hours of lecture and laboratory work, and possibly some small group discussions.

A newer approach employed by some schools replaced the discipline-based curriculum with one organized on an interdisciplinary, organ system basis. In this type of curriculum, students study all aspects of each organ system before moving on to the next. Instruction is interdisciplinary, with faculty members from many departments forming teaching teams. Proponents of this approach believe that the organ system model provides better integration of the material to be learned.

Some schools use a hybrid of the two traditional curricular models. For example, the first year may be organized with traditional, discipline-based courses, while the second employs the interdisciplinary organ system approach. Or, elements of both may be mixed during parts of the curriculum.

Problem-Based Learning

A relatively new arrival on the medical education scene is Problem-Based Learning (PBL). In PBL, case-oriented problems are reviewed by small groups of medical students working together as a team under the direction of a faculty member. The PBL teams review the case material presented, identify learning issues, and assign those issues to group members. Each group member researches the issue assigned and reports back to the group at a subsequent meeting. As the cases unravel, the students not only begin to learn the basics of clinical medicine (the vocabulary, normal lab values, etcetera), but they're challenged to understand the basic physiology, pathology, and pharmacology of the disease as well.

Some medical schools employ PBL almost exclusively. Others use PBL in conjunction with more traditional approaches, selecting the best approach for the material to be covered. The latter schools endeavor to coordinate the PBL cases with material covered in the traditional courses.

Earliest Patient Contact

There is a trend toward providing patient contact early in the curriculum, often as early as the first few weeks of the first year. Proponents of this argue that medical students will find their studies more meaningful if they are combined with the chance to work with patients right from the start of medical school. Those who advocate delaying such contact point out that students can do little but observe until they have obtained enough training to be of real help to their patients. Medical schools differ as to when and how they provide this contact.

Organization of the Clinical Years

The third and fourth years of medical school are designed to equip you with the knowledge, skills, attitudes, and behaviors necessary for further training in medicine. This is done by providing you with clinical experiences in a variety of clinical settings. You can expect some exposure to family medicine, internal medicine, obstetrics and gynecology, pediatrics, psychiatry, and surgery. Some schools will require you to complete these core experiences, called clerkships, before moving on to other areas of medicine. Other schools will provide more flexibility in scheduling and may permit some electives or selectives throughout the third and fourth years. Schools will also differ in the extent to which they will permit off-campus, and even international, electives during the clinical years.

Primary Care Focus

Some medical schools clearly state that their mission is to increase the number of primary care (family practice, general internal medicine, general pediatrics, and possibly obstetrics and gynecology) physicians in practice. These schools structure their curricula to emphasize opportunities in primary care and may attempt to select applicants who show a higher likelihood of entering primary care specialties.

Innovative Educational Approaches

Medical education is evolving rapidly and new approaches are being tried at many schools. Computer-assisted instruction is widely utilized and some schools now require entering students to own their own computer. Simulated patients are used by many schools to help students learn to conduct patient interviews and to examine patients. Self instruction, also referred to as self-directed learning, is emphasized in many schools. New methodologies are being developed regularly.

Student Evaluation and Grading

An essential component to the curriculum is the method by which you will be evaluated. One way in which medical schools differ is in the grading system employed. Grading systems can vary from a simple pass-fail system to a five-step system, such as A-B-C-D-F. Others use a numerical system. A three-point system of Honors-Pass-Fail is common. Some schools use different systems for different parts of the curriculum, such as Honors-Pass-Fail for required courses, and Pass-Fail for electives. Some schools will employ Objective Structured Clinical Examinations (OSCE) during the clinical years.

United States Medical Licensing Examination Policies

The USMLE is the series of examinations required of all applicants for a medical license in any state in the United States. The USMLE is actually made up of three steps. Step 1 is usually taken at the end of the second year of medical school, Step 2 during the senior year, and Step 3 at the end of the first year of residency. The majority of medical schools require their students to pass Step 1 to be promoted to the third year or to graduate. Many schools also require Step 2 passage for graduation. Some residency programs also consider your scores on Step 1 when you apply for residency.

Special Programs and Opportunities

One of the ways in which medical schools differentiate themselves is with the special programs they offer. These may be in the form of research opportunities, opportunities for community involvement, international educational experiences, or in any number of other ways too numerous to mention.

These are all important issues for you to consider. Be sure to consult school Web pages, request catalogs, and review the MSAR to find out what approach is used at the schools you're interested in. Another resource is the AAMC Curriculum Directory, available from the same place you order the MSAR. Do your research! You should know how the schools you're interested in differ in each of the ways discussed. Weigh the pros and cons of each factor and decide which is most appropriate for your learning style. Remember, each medical school will ask you to articulate why you have chosen it.

Teaching Hospitals

Just as important as the basic science curriculum that a medical school offers is its affiliated teaching hospitals. You'll be doing your clinical rotations predominantly in those hospitals and clinics that are designated as teaching hospitals of that school. Your first clinical experiences will be shaped, in large part, by the types of hospitals to which you are exposed. For example, if a medical school is primarily associated with city hospitals, you'll probably be exposed to a disproportionate amount of trauma and emergency medicine. Likewise, if Veteran Administration hospitals predominate, you may encounter many cases of emphysema, heart disease, and posttraumatic stress disorder. What you experience during your clinical rotations may greatly influence your choice of specialty.

Location

Location is another important consideration in deciding where to apply to medical school. Most premedical students, however, are so concerned about whether or not they'll be accepted by any school that they fail to consider if they'll be happy spending four years in that locale. Applicants tend to evaluate the medical schools lists based on reputation and prestige, rather than location and lifestyle. Don't make this mistake. The bottom line is that you should choose a school where you'll be happy and comfortable for four years. Medical school has enough stresses with the long hours and hard work. Don't complicate matters by choosing a school in a place where day-to-day living will be a chore.

Take the following location-related factors into account when making your choice:

Safety

Many medical centers are located in inner cities with associated high rates of crime. It's obviously an added stress to be in an area in which you feel unsafe. Some medical centers will provide escorts and other security services. Keep this in mind when you're visiting schools and inquire about safety issues. If you're really concerned, you can call the local police station and ask for crime statistics.

Housing

Remember that in addition to tuition, you'll also have to pay for housing, food, and transportation. Unfortunately, due to the location of some schools, nearby housing is either unsafe or unaffordable. In some inner-city schools, the majority of the student body resides in dormitories. These dorms are often expensive and have inadequate kitchen facilities. Nonetheless, they may be the best alternatives given the medical school's location.

In contrast, students who decide to attend equally good programs that are based in small towns or communities may be pleasantly surprised to find inexpensive housing near the school. Crime will not be as big a problem in these areas.

Transportation

This is obviously important as it pertains to housing and community shops. If there isn't housing near the medical center or its affiliated hospitals, then you'll need to have a car. If you don't, it is important that there be adequate public transportation, whether it be a bus line or subway system.

Proximity to Family and Friends

If there are special people in your life with whom you enjoy spending time, it may be important for you to live nearby. Medical school does not afford you much free time, and the time it takes to travel can easily make frequent or lengthy visits difficult.

Affiliation with an Undergraduate Institution

It's of great benefit to you if your medical school is part of a larger institution. Typically, the undergraduate institution allows the graduate students to enjoy the same privileges as the undergrads. This will include gym facilities, movies, libraries, clubs, and other organizations. In addition, if the institution has strong athletic teams, then graduate students have access to tickets and can enjoy this diversion from class work.

Student Body

Some schools are known for having a competitive atmosphere, in which students feel little camaraderie with one another. At other schools, a sense of "We're all in it together" prevails. Think about how much

> ### *Read All about It*
>
> If you're considering a particular locale, get your hands on its newspaper. This will give you a handle on the cost of living, available transportation, and local issues.

the attitude of other students matters to you. You can probably get a sense of a school's "flavor" by visiting schools or asking your premed advisor.

You may also want to find out about schools' gender and ethnic balances. While many schools strive to create a diverse student body, some are more diligent in their efforts than others. Check our school profiles in the appendix as well as your MSAR for the particulars.

Public versus Private Schools

For most students, the best chance for admission is at a public medical school located in their home state. This is because public medical schools give strong preference in admission to their own residents. In addition, some private schools give at least a little admissions preference to residents of the state in which they are located. As a result, according to AAMC statistics, 67.7 percent of the students who entered medical school in 1999 enrolled in schools in their home state. For this reason, you should take a close look at schools located in your home state as you consider schools to which you will apply.

While a few private schools give some preference to in-state applicants, most do not. Since the majority of applicants apply to at least some private schools the result is that most private schools receive large numbers of applications, sometimes over 10,000, for an entering class size of less than 200 students. Don't let these high numbers discourage you, though, because they are the result of multiple applications. In 1999, the average applicant applied to 11.5 schools. In other words, many of the same people apply to the same schools.

Unless you are an exceptionally strong candidate, your chances of gaining admission to a public school

located outside your home state are relatively small. Since most public schools give preference to in-state applicants, (some are prohibited from admitting nonresidents), the competition for admission to these schools as a nonresident is very keen. On the other hand, a few public schools will admit a reasonable number of nonresidents. In 1998, 16 public schools enrolled at least 15 percent nonresidents, and 10 enrolled 20 percent or more. If you are a very strong applicant and have an interest in a particular public school you should consult that school's admissions office for advice.

The individual school entries in the MSAR describe the school's residency preferences and list the number of applicants and matriculants by residency status. This is an excellent place to start looking for schools that might consider you.

Early Decision Program (EDP)

A little more than half of the medical schools in the United States offer early decision programs. For an EDP, you file only one application to the one medical school you wish to attend. Most schools accept these special applications around mid-June. You are prohibited from applying to any other schools until the school has rendered a decision. If you're accepted, then you must attend. Most schools notify candidates by October 1.

Early decision programs are appropriate only for very competitive applicants who have a strong preference for one particular school. These applicants benefit in that they save considerable money on applications, interviews, and travel. In addition, they know where they're going to med school by October.

> ### First Choice, Only Choice
>
> Apply early decision only if you feel strongly about your first choice, and only if you're certain that if you're accepted you'll attend. If you apply early decision but don't get in, you'll be playing application catch-up.

If you apply early decision but are not accepted, you'll be behind your peers in the application process. It's not a decision—or a possible consequence—to be taken lightly. You should definitely sit down with your premed advisor and decide if this option is appropriate for you.

Different But Equal: Osteopathic Physician

Doctor of Osteopathy degrees are virtually indistinguishable in practice from medical doctor degrees. D.O.'s work alongside M.D.'s or in their own practices. Like allopathic medical school, the osteopathic course of study spans four years: two years of basic education and two years of clinical rotations. After the degree is obtained, D.O.'s also complete residency. Osteopathic medicine more typically focuses on the whole person, leading D.O.'s to practice more often in primary care fields, such as internal medicine, family practice, and pediatrics. They are licensed to prescribe medicine, and they can admit patients to hospitals.

The difference between allopathic and osteopathic practice lies in focus and reputation. Osteopaths believe that a problem in one body part will cause distress in another. In addition, according to osteopathic medicine, the body can regulate and heal itself if conditions allow for it to do so. The biggest obstacle to this healing process is physical or emotional stress. To osteopaths, musculoskeletal health is key to preventing and overcoming illness and disease. By treating the musculoskeletal system, the disease cycle can be interrupted. Osteopathic medicine focuses on relaxation of muscles, tendons, and connective tissue.

Humane Medical Philosophy

"You get the same training as an M.D. in osteopathic school, as well as additional training in muscular and skeletal manipulation, and alternative forms of treatment. D.O.'s can go into M.D. residencies, prescribe drugs, and perform surgery. I also think osteopathy is a more humane medical philosophy, treating a patient as a patient, not as a disease."

—D.O., University of New England

Although osteopaths are highly regarded, especially as the United States focuses on primary health care needs, a D.O. degree may make it slightly more difficult to get a highly competitive residency. It is also more competitive to get into osteopathic schools: Fewer than one in five applicants is accepted.

The *College Information Booklet* gives a brief description of each of the 19 osteopathic medical colleges, including admissions criteria, minimum entrance requirements, supplementary application materials required, class size or enrollment, application deadlines, and tuition. A single copy costs $2.00 and may be ordered by sending a check or money order (including 20 percent for postage and handling) to:

American Association of Colleges of Osteopathic Medicine–AACOM
5550 Friendship Boulevard, Suite 310
Chevy Chase, MD 20815-7231
(301) 968-4100
www.aacom.org

CHAPTER 5

Researching Medical Schools

Though it may be tempting to apply to schools without having researched them, succumbing to this temptation may get you into trouble later in the process. Medical school admissions committees are most interested in an applicant whose decision to apply to their school is clearly an informed one. You should demonstrate enough specific interest in the school that the committee believes you would accept its offer over one from another school.

The goal of your information gathering is not just to formulate a list of medical schools for the general AMCAS application, but to be able to take each medical school on your list and cite several specific reasons you have decided to apply there (and not just "Well, it's in the top twenty" or "I think I can get in"). This approach will serve you well at two important points in the application process: secondary applications and interviews.

Variations on the question, "Why have you decided to apply here?" appear in many secondary applications. This is the admissions committee's first attempt to plumb the depths of your motivation to go not just to medical school, but to its medical school. A strong statement of reasons you're enthusiastic about the school will immediately put your application in a more favorable light. If you're informed, you can write at length about what specifically attracts you about the school: its innovative curriculum, the emphasis on problem-based learning, the opportunities to spend time doing research with famous professors X and Y, to spend an elective abroad in India, etcetera.

Researching a particular medical school and being able to make a strong argument about why you and the school are a good match can help you with that school's secondary application. It can also help you during the interview. There are numerous ways to find out everything you want to know about medical schools. They range from official AAMC-produced publications, to commercial and online sources, to word of mouth.

Westward, Ho!

WICHE, the Western Interstate Commission for Higher Education, has a professional exchange program, in which medical students from Alaska, Montana, and Wyoming can attend participating western schools (all but the University of Washington participate) and pay in-state tuition. For more information, contact WICHE:

Professional Student Exchange Program
Western Interstate Commission for Higher Education
P.O. Box 9752
Boulder, CO 80301-9752
tel: (303) 541-0210
www.wiche.edu

Milking the MSAR

As we said in chapter 4, it's worth your while to order your own copy of the MSAR from the AAMC as soon as you get a chance. The MSAR is as close as you can get to a premed bible, especially considering the fact that the information it contains on all of the medical schools comes directly from the schools themselves. The book is divided into two main parts: admission information and school profiles.

Part 1: Admissions

The first part of the MSAR is entitled "Admission Information." Be sure to read through all of it carefully; there are about one hundred pages of important information about the admissions process here. For example, look at Table 5A in chapter 5. It shows just how much a school's admissions decisions are affected by whether or not the school receives funding from its state government. It may tell you, for example, that only 29 percent of the applicants to School X are residents of the state School X is located in, but 91 percent of the new entrants are state residents. Clearly the admissions committee of School X gave a lot of preference to state residents, in all likelihood because this has been required of them in return for state funding. Some medical schools even have quotas for specific regions of the state. They may accept more people from underserved areas of the state in the hope that these applicants will go back and practice medicine in the communities in which they were raised.

If you were a resident of School X's state, you would naturally be very happy about this, but if you weren't, you would know from the information on this table that you would have to be extremely qualified to be accepted as one of that last 9 percent. (At some state schools you are likely be admitted only if you plan to do an M.D./Ph.D. or if you are a member of an underrepresented minority.)

Take note of one thing about this table, though: Percent of new entrants is not the same thing as percent of applicants accepted. The percentage of accepted applicants that were in-state could have been a bit higher or lower than the percentage of new entrants that were in-state.

Part 2: Profiles

The second part of the MSAR contains profiles of all the accredited schools in the United States and Canada. Each school packs a lot of info into its allotted two pages. Here's a breakdown of what you can expect to find in each profile.

General Information

Medical schools use this section to describe themselves, their history, their physical facilities, and affiliated teaching hospitals. They will indicate whether the school is public or private.

Curriculum

The curricula of many medical schools have undergone or are undergoing major change; the trend is toward some degree of incorporation of problem-based learning into the curriculum. In this section, the medical school typically outlines the different components of its curriculum, including the progression of courses over the first two years, the exposure to clinical medicine, and electives. The school may offer more than one curriculum, and often the school's M.D./Ph.D. option is mentioned here.

Native Tongues

The three Puerto Rican med schools require proficiency in Spanish, while three of Canada's 16 accredited med schools conduct courses in French.

Requirements for Entrance

While this section generally holds few surprises regarding prerequisite course work and test taking (the MCAT), requirements can vary a little from school to school. For example, for the 1999 entering class, there were 80 schools that had a one-year English requirement, while 17 schools required a year of humanities. Skip this section at your own risk; you might not have fulfilled all of the requirements for your dream school.

Sometimes an admissions committee will go out of its way to assert that it will consider applicants who have majored in any field as long as the work done in that major was exemplary. Some schools even state that they do not give any preference to those who majored in the sciences. Good news, if you're an English or history major.

Selection Factors

Look here for important data such as the mean GPA and MCAT scores for the most recent entering class, the distribution of applicants or entrants by undergraduate major or school, the mean age of students, and the percentage of women and minorities in the entering class. Many schools will not disclose their numerical criteria for selection, since they make an effort to judge students as individuals, not as numbers.

Your GPA and MCAT scores are by no means the only factors that go into an admissions committee's decision, and most schools take the opportunity here to sketch out the qualities they like to see in an applicant. However, the numbers they publish for GPA and MCAT can be used as a crude indicator of how competitive a school is to get into. A school whose students have a mean GPA of 3.6 and double-digit MCAT scores is probably more competitive than a school whose students have a mean GPA of 3.3 and a mean MCAT score of 8.

If a school systematically gives preference based on geography, whether it be to in-state applicants only or to applicants from nearby states as well (as is the case with the University of Washington at Seattle), you should find a statement to that effect in the "Selection Factors" section.

Financial Aid

In this section, schools give a brief description of their resources in terms of scholarships and loans available to medical students. Often a school will also indicate the percentage of the student body that receives financial aid. (Note: When you decide which medical school to attend, you should work closely with that school's financial aid office. You'd be surprised at the number of loans, grants, scholarships, and fellowships that are available.)

Several points come up fairly often in the "Financial Aid" section of the school profiles:

- Some schools state a preference that their students not be otherwise employed while in school.
- Non-U.S. citizens without permanent resident or visa status are not eligible to receive financial aid, and often must be able to prove their ability to pay.
- Many assert that financial need has no bearing on whether an applicant will be accepted.

Information for Minorities

A quick survey across medical schools in this section shows the depth of commitment the schools have to the active recruitment of underrepresented minority and disadvantaged applicants. Many schools have offerings designed to support and encourage such applicants, including loans, scholarships, and postbaccalaureate and prematricular programs.

Admissions committees typically have significant minority representation, and most medical schools have personnel such as minority student advisers or minority recruitment coordinators who can provide guidance and information for minority applicants.

Application and Acceptance Policies

This section of the school profile provides you with some key pieces of information:

AMCAS Deadline

Traditionally, all AMCAS schools have one of the following deadlines: October 15, November 1, November 15, December 1, or December 15.

School Application Fee

Be aware that this refers to the fee you will have to pay in addition to the AMCAS fee. Most schools require you to pay this fee when you submit their secondary applications. Pay attention to the way the school application fee is listed. You can infer from information here whether a school does an initial review of your application before they send you a secondary application. Some schools have an "application fee to all applicants"; other schools, including the University of California programs, say that they charge an application fee after "screening." Those in the latter category will be doing an initial review of your application before they send you a secondary application and request the application fee. If you apply and receive a secondary application from such a school, you can give yourself a pat on the back for making the first cut.

Oldest Acceptable MCAT Scores

Schools vary widely in their willingness to accept old scores, so if you took the MCAT a couple of years ago but have held off on applying, you should look at this closely—you may have to retake the MCAT to get into the school of your choice. Most schools will take scores that are two or three years old, but a few will accept only scores received in the four administrations immediately preceding entry into schools.

Early Decision Program Deadlines

As we described in the last chapter, slightly more than half of the medical schools in the United States offer early decision programs. With early decision, you file only one application to the one medical school you wish to attend. You can't apply to any other school until the EDP school has rendered a decision on your application. If you're accepted, you must attend. Most schools notify the candidates of their decision by October 1.

Other Elements

This section of the MSAR also contains:

- Earliest dates for acceptance notices
- Availability of option to defer
- Amount of deposit to hold place in class
- Estimated number of new entrants
- Starting date of classes

Information on Previous Year's Classes

Here is yet another opportunity to figure out how partial a school is to in-state residents, since two sets of numbers (in-state and out-of-state) are given for the categories of "number of applicants," "number of applicants interviewed," and "new entrants."

This section also serves as a very general barometer of how difficult it is for an applicant to obtain admission to the school, since you can use the numbers to calculate the percentage of applicants that are granted interviews and the percentage of those granted interviews who are actually admitted. One caveat, however: You have to take into account the fact that one school's applicant pool may well be stronger than another's if you are trying to compare them. If Harvard and Podunk U. Med both take five percent of their applicants, this clearly does not mean that they are equally competitive.

The Rankings

You've probably heard about the rankings of medical schools in *U.S. News & World Report*. These rankings do indeed contain some valuable information, such as:

- Amount of NIH-funded research for each school
- Faculty-to-student ratio
- Out-of-state tuition
- Percentage of graduates that have gone into primary care fields

From the rankings, you can also get a pretty good sense of how prestigious schools are as well as how difficult they are to get into. This information can be useful when you are formulating your overall application strategy and trying to determine your particular "dream" and "safety" schools.

Take rankings with a grain of salt, however, because they are pretty subjective. Make sure you read the explanations of the methodology employed in putting each ranking together so that you understand exactly what you are getting. You should also review rankings from previous years in order to see how they and their underlying methodologies have recently changed.

Of course, rankings leave out a lot of important information. They tell you nothing about how well a particular school treats its students as a whole (this does vary from school to school), what the professors and the students are like, what special offerings the school's curriculum might have, or what the social life and housing arrangements are like. You shouldn't assume that a school's high ranking automatically means it would be a good choice for you.

Hospital Rankings

In addition to its yearly rankings of medical schools, *U.S. News & World Report* also publishes rankings of hospitals affiliated with medical schools (you can find these in a separate issue entitled *America's Best*

Hospitals). The rankings go specialty by specialty, so you'll find them particularly useful if you already have an interest in a specific branch of medicine. The teaching hospitals are, after all, where you will be receiving your clinical training during your clerkships (the third and fourth years at almost every medical school).

The rankings include information on:

- Hospital reputation
- Mortality rate (for specialties for which this is applicable)
- Number of residents, doctors, nurses, and inpatient operations to beds
- Number of high-tech services available

On-Campus Sources

Visiting a med school you're considering attending or asking around the university you currently attend can give you great insight into a school's particular flavor, including the kind of student who's been accepted in the med school. Med students, grad students, undergrads, and faculty can all shed light on your chances of admission—and of your potential happiness at a particular medical school.

> **Inside Scoop**
>
> Ask current med students about the schools they attend and how they got in. Not only will you get info on what worked for them in the application process, but you'll also get a sense of whether a particular school is right for you.

Med Students

If you attend a university that has a medical school, you're in luck; you can't help but get an idea of what the medical program is like, and you may well have some contact with the med students, even if this is only because they sometimes eat at the same cafeteria you do. Ask them how they got accepted to medical school, what they did as an undergraduate, where else they applied to (and were accepted or rejected). They've been through the process; they've already done the information gathering, the applications, the interviews, and the financial aid forms. No doubt they're proud of being accepted to med school, and you know how willing people are to discuss their achievements. You'll learn things about the medical schools that you could never pick up from a book.

Ph.D. Students

In addition, universities with medical schools typically have affiliated programs that grant Ph.D.'s in the biomedical sciences. Ph.D. students often will not hesitate to comment on their own program (you may be interested in doing an M.D./Ph.D.), their professors (who may also be on the medical school faculty), the research at the university, and the medical students.

Premed Seniors

If you are not so fortunate as to have a medical school nearby (and even if you do), be sure to seek advice from the premed seniors at your college before they graduate. They have gone through the process of applying and are interviewing and making their decisions as the school year progresses. They will be an extremely good source of up-to-date information about the medical schools; after all, the admissions process has taken up a considerable amount of their time and mental energy in the past year.

Your Premed Adviser

As mentioned earlier, don't underestimate the importance of premed advisers as a source of information about medical schools. Advisers who have held their positions for a substantial period of time have built up links and personal contacts with admissions personnel at different medical schools—which means they have gotten feedback from them in one form or another about applicants they sent to them in the past. They know which schools may overlook a disastrous freshman year if they see a trend of improvement; which schools will accept large numbers of nontraditional students (that is, older students changing careers); which schools are known to give sons and daughters of alumni and faculty preferential treatment; and, most important, which medical schools like to accept students from your college or university.

Premed advisers are also the individuals best suited to give you the information you may want—more than anything else—about a particular school: your chances of getting in. They can roughly judge how competitive you will be as an applicant because they have already advised students with your approximate profile (GPA, MCATs, extracurriculars) and they know how these previous applicants have fared. They may even have compiled statistics on those who have gone before you in order to help make such evaluations. Of course, bear in mind that you are a unique candidate and your premed adviser is not the one making the admissions decisions.

The typical premed advisory office also has a wealth of information in the form of catalogs, brochures, and announcements. They may also have videos on the AAMC and on some of the medical schools.

Catalogs

Reading med school catalogs can give you great insight into the specifics of a school. You should carefully read the catalog for each school to which you're applying. The admissions committee will expect you to have read the school's catalog before you complete the secondary application—certainly before you show up for the interview.

Order your catalogs from the schools you're thinking about applying to in the late spring, before you start working on the AMCAS application; that way, you'll beat the rush. (Some schools may not be ready with their new catalogs yet, but you'll get on their back-order list.) To request catalogs, call the admissions office numbers listed in the appendix; in most cases you'll just have to leave your name and number on an answering machine.

Reading the Catalog

Keep in mind that the medical school catalog is a marketing tool as well as a repository of information. Schools are interested in attracting the best students they can, so they put their best foot forward. (Undergraduate schools do the same thing, of course; take a look at the current catalog or brochure your undergraduate institution puts out and compare it with your personal experience.) Take the catalog photos with a grain of salt: Though they can provide some valuable information, a good photographer can make a medical center situated in the middle of an urban war zone look like a country club.

Many catalogs also profile some of the school's students, describing their educational background, their extracurricular activities in college and at the medical school, the offices they hold in medical student organizations, and their career plans. While the students profiled are outstanding in some way or another, they are not necessarily representative of the average student at the school. Never decide that you will not be a competitive applicant at a school just because you didn't spend two years deep in the heart of Brazil learning about the medicinal properties of rare plants from the natives like the student profiled in the school's catalog did.

Glossy photos and student profiles notwithstanding, the catalog does contain a lot of information that is not only necessary to know for interviews but will also help you compare that school to others you are interested in. Here are some things to look for.

Educational Priorities

Schools differ in their emphasis on primary care versus research/specialization. The current trend is to encourage greater numbers of graduates to go into primary care, since there is a recognized shortage of primary care physicians and a relative overabundance of specialists in this country. However, some schools with a long tradition of producing leaders in research and academic medicine continue to recognize their responsibility for training the next generation of biomedical scientists.

> ### *Research versus Service*
>
> Even heavy research schools value a diverse student body, so don't hesitate to express a commitment to public service to a school known for its excellence in research.

Once you have read and compared a few catalogs, you will be able to discern each catalog's underlying message concerning the school's educational priorities. One catalog will spend a single paragraph on "Research Opportunities" but boast right in the introduction that over 45 percent of the graduates do their residencies in primary care. Another will devote pages and pages to the "Special Study and Research Experiences" available and go on at great length about the amount of NIH funding the Nobel laureates on the faculty receive yearly. Considering this, it's not hard to tell where each school stands. Catalogs will be especially useful in determining the general educational orientation of the many schools that do not appear on the commercial lists.

Application Requirements

The section on requirements is another chance for you to make sure that you've taken all of the courses required by a school, and that your application contains all the necessary components. Read any information concerning letters of recommendation very carefully. You're usually safe with admissions committees if you are submitting a packet of letters or a composite letter from your undergraduate school's preprofessional committee. If you're not, though, each medical school has specific requirements about the number and distribution (in terms of academic departments) of recommendations they want you to send them, and these requirements do vary from school to school. Also, if you have been away from your undergraduate school for some time, you may be expected to submit recommendations from employers or graduate school professors. Ask your premedical adviser if you have any questions about recommendation letters; he or she has handled this issue with many students before.

Where Students Come From, Where They're Going

Matchmaker, Matchmaker

A statistic many schools cite is the percentage of students who match at one of their top-three residency choices. The "match" is a process by which senior med students and residency programs rank each other. A computer program then matches a student with a residency program. It's prestigious for a school to have a high percentage (>85 percent) of their students match at their first choice of residencies.

Many medical schools list their recent graduates and where those graduates are doing their residencies; some also give statistics on where their first-year students went to college. The list of residencies gives you a general indication of the reputation of the medical school among residency directors, and you can compare the relative success of students from different schools (you will probably want to ask a medical student or doctor whom you know or consult *U.S. News'* "Best Hospitals" issue to determine the reputation of the teaching hospitals where the graduates are doing their residencies). Information about the first-year students' undergraduate school of origin may be important since a medical school's admissions committee may well have had favorable results with accepting students from your college in the past, and, therefore, be that much more willing to consider your application.

Curriculum

Every medical school catalog contains a detailed description of the curriculum (some have graphs that lay the whole four years out for you very nicely). Take note of any changes that have been made in the past few years, such as earlier exposure to patients and the institution of problem-based learning. You will also find information about combined-degree programs, electives you can spend abroad, research tracks, and other special opportunities.

No doubt you'll be interested in how students are evaluated in their coursework and whether or not you'll be ranked numerically within your class; this will be in the catalog as well.

Faculty and Their Research

Not all schools list their faculty in the catalog, but if they do, you can look up the names of faculty members in the field or department you are interested in and then do an online or CD-ROM search of MEDLINE, the medical journal database, to read about the research they have published recently. This is particularly important to do if you are applying to combined-degree programs and plan to do research as part of your medical education.

Student Resources and Services

How are the school's libraries and computer resources, recreation facilities, and student health service? Can you find decent, affordable housing in the area, and what help will the school give you in your search? If the school is located in a dangerous part of town, is there a student shuttle to take you where you want to go? What about guidance on course selection and career planning? The school catalog can provide at least partial answers to these and other practical questions. (You may have to wait until you visit the campus for the interview to get the whole picture, but catalogs often provide the addresses and telephone numbers of the school housing office, the libraries, and other resources that will help get you started.)

Student Organizations

Medical schools like to accept individuals who have been involved in extracurricular, community, and volunteer activities, so it's no surprise that they typically offer a wide range of student organizations and activities. If you read about an organization or an activity in the catalog that appeals to you, tell the admissions committee about your interest, especially if you have something in your background to suggest that you would truly be committed to it. If you were deeply involved in student government in college, for example, and would want to continue by serving in medical student government, let them know.

Valuable Info

MEDLINE is a database, operated by the National Library of Medicine, that houses information on medical and health journals, books, and other publications. You can use it to search for clinical information, research news, and health updates. You can get more information on MEDLINE by calling: (888) FIND-NLM.

Or surf the NLM's Web site: http://www.nlm.nih.gov.

The World Wide Web

The amount of medical school information that can be retrieved from the Web is already truly staggering, and it will only increase in the future. Almost every medical school has a home page; once you're there, you'll find out everything you could have gotten from the catalog—and more. In addition, you can use the Web to learn more about the professors in your research field at each school, to read the insights and advice of medical students who have made it through the process, and to prepare for interviews by perusing the comments of former interviewees at different schools.

Kaplan Online

Check out Kaplan's sites for up-to-the-minute info on test prep, admissions, and financial aid:

- America Online: Keyword "Kaplan"
- World Wide Web: http://www.kaptest.com

Use your Web browser to search for sites by using "medical school" or the name of the school you want to learn more about as the search words, and you'll be off and running. Bear in mind that the Web is constantly changing, so browse often.

A word of caution: WYSIWYG. What you see is what you get. Keep in mind that while most of the information you get from the Web can be extremely helpful, some of it may be incomplete or inaccurate. For example, admissions advice from a medical student may only reflect that student's personal experience and may not accurately reflect how the admissions process works at all medical schools.

Making Your List and Checking it Twice . . .

Now comes the fun part: making your list. As you begin selecting the schools you will be applying to, keep in mind everything you learned poring over medical school catalogs, learning the MSAR by heart, studying this chapter, and listening to the sage advice of your premed adviser. While everyone should have a few schools that constitute a "wish list" (Hey, it could happen!), you basically have to remember to use your head when you select to which schools to apply. Remember that more is not necessarily better, but it is more expensive.

PART FOUR

Getting In

CHAPTER 6

Meeting Admissions Requirements

Unlike the college application process, which you started in the fall or, for late bloomers, in the early winter of your senior year of high school, the medical school application process starts considerably earlier. Why? Because there is much more to do and, with the odds of getting accepted to any school being quite low, more preparation is necessary. You can't just wake up one morning and decide to apply to medical school this year. Med schools have a whole set of prerequisites for admission that you may not yet have taken as an undergraduate.

> **Focus**
>
> Throughout the application process, focus on what you can learn from the experience, not just what you can do to get into medical school. Doing so will help you keep your goals in sight.

Researching med schools early in the process means knowing exactly what courses you need to take before you apply. You'll also learn what courses you can take during the 18-month application period, as well as what courses you should have completed before you take the Medical College Admission Test (MCAT). Since some courses are both grueling and key to getting accepted, you can plan to avoid taking, say, organic chemistry and calculus simultaneously.

Specific Course Requirements

Nearly all schools require work in the biological sciences, chemistry (general and organic) and physics. About two-thirds of the schools require English and about 25 percent require calculus. A small number of schools have no specific course requirements. Bear in mind, however, that since the MCAT covers material from the commonly required courses, you will need to include those courses in your program of study whether they are required by medical schools or not. Nevertheless, many students are surprised to learn that the list of courses required by medical schools is so small.

The best sources for specific information on prerequisites are the *Medical School Admission Requirements* (MSAR), which lists requirements for all accredited allopathic medical schools, and the *College Information Booklet,* which contains similar information on all of the country's osteopathic medical schools. These publications will also tell you of each school's other admission requirements such as minimum semester hours required and whether a bachelor's degree is essential.

Beyond the Requirements

Since the list of courses required by medical schools is short, you will need to decide what else to take. Many of your decisions will be governed by the requirements of the major and degree you are seeking. Even so, you will probably be faced with at least some choices every semester or quarter. You will need to choose specific courses within your major and you will have to select various electives.

According to the AAMC, 1998 medical school graduates who were asked to rate the importance of undergraduate courses they had taken to their medical school experiences ranked physiology as the most important subject. Others named as important (besides the required courses) included biochemistry, advanced biology, genetics, comparative anatomy, and English composition. A number of additional subjects ranging from advanced organic chemistry to psychology and English composition were found to be of some value by those who had taken them. Interestingly, calculus was taken by a very large majority of the students but those students cited it as not at all important to their medical studies.

How to choose? One approach is to broaden your education by considering at least some social science and humanities electives if you are a science major. Conversely, if you are a nonscience major, consider taking at least some additional science courses. Think about the subjects medical graduates found to be helpful, but don't try to take all of them. Remember, the important thing is that you gain a broad, well-rounded education, keeping in mind that your undergraduate education will be your foundation for your entire life, not just medical school. Finally, to the extent possible, take courses that interest you. You will do better and have a more enjoyable time.

The MCAT

For nearly all schools, the MCAT carries significant weight in the admissions process. Administered by the Association of American Medical Colleges, the MCAT is a relatively objective way to compare you with other applicants. Medical schools use MCAT scores to assess whether you have the foundation upon which to build a successful medical career. Though it's hard to believe that a single test could indicate how good a doctor you'll be, the evidence seems to indicate that the MCAT does predict how good a medical student you'll be: A November 1996 article in the journal *Academic Medicine* concluded that MCAT scores are an excellent indicator of success in med school and on the medical boards. Though that's not the final word on your future medical competency, it does give medical admissions committees a way to approximate your potential in the medical arena.

The MCAT is not a straightforward science test; it's a thinking test. This means that the test is designed to let you demonstrate not only your breadth of knowledge, but your thought processes as well.

What's On the Test

The MCAT consists of four sections: Verbal Reasoning, Physical Sciences, Writing Sample, and Biological Sciences. There are five and three-quarter hours of testing, including multiple-choice questions and two essays. Add in the two ten-minute breaks, one hour for lunch, and some time for administrivia, and you're talking about a seven- to eight-hour day of testing.

Breaking it down into parts, here's how you'll spend your day.

Morning:

Verbal Reasoning

Time:	85 minutes
Format:	65 multiple-choice questions; approximately 9–10 passages with 6–10 questions each
What it tests:	critical reading

(10-minute break)

Physical Science

Time:	100 minutes
Format:	77 multiple-choice questions; approximately 10–11 passages with 4–8 questions each; 15 stand-alone questions (not passage based)
What it tests:	basic general-chemistry concepts; basic physics concepts; analytical reasoning; data interpretation

(Lunch: 60-minute break)

Writing Sample

Time:	60 minutes
Format:	2 essay questions (30 minutes per essay)
What it tests:	critical thinking; intellectual organization; written communication skills

(Afternoon: 10-minute break)

Biological Sciences

Time:	100 minutes
Format:	77 multiple-choice questions; approximately 10–11 passages with 4–8 questions each; 15 stand-alone questions (not passage-based)
What it tests:	basic biology concepts; basic organic chemistry concepts; analytical reasoning; data interpretation

How It's Scored

Each section has its own score. The scores in the Verbal Reasoning, Physical Sciences, and Biological Sciences sections range from 1–15. The Writing Sample score will be a letter from J to T (basically an 11-point range). Each of the two essays you write are evaluated by two official readers; the four critiques are combined to yield your alphabetical score. All of the multiple-choice questions have the same value, and the number of your correct answers is converted into a "scaled" score and a percentile (how you did relative to everyone else who took the exam).

The average scaled score for each test is about 8 for the numbered tests and about N for the writing sample. What's a good score? Well, with the competition so fierce, you'll want to aim for at least 10 or 11 (12 and above for the top schools).

That's not to say you won't get in somewhere with a lower score. Bear in mind that schools report the average MCAT score of their students. So a school reporting an average of 10 clearly means that plenty of the students scored 10 or lower. However, the range of MCAT scores for accepted applicants for a given school is typically rather narrow. In other words, if a med school's average accepted MCAT score is 10, you're not going to see many 7's and 8's.

You'll get four different scores for the four sections. If you aced one or two sections but fell a bit in one or two others, your total score will still look pretty good.

You don't have to be perfect to do well. On a recent MCAT administration, you could get as many as 4 questions wrong in Verbal Reasoning, 21 in Physical Sciences, and 16 in Biological Sciences and still score in the eightieth percentile. To score in the ninetieth percentile, you could get as many as 2 wrong in Verbal Reasoning, 16 in Physical Sciences, and 11 in Biological Sciences. Even students who receive perfect scaled scores usually get a handful of questions wrong.

It's important to maximize your performance on every question. Just a few questions one way or the other can make a big difference in your scaled score. Here's a look at recent score profiles so you can get an idea of the shape of a typical score distribution.

Verbal Reasoning

Scaled Score	Percent Achieving Score	Percentile Rank Range
13–15	01.0	99.1–99.9
12	03.4	95.7–99.0
11	10.7	85.0–95.6
10	15.1	69.9–84.9
9	18.7	51.2–69.8
8	13.1	38.1–51.1
7	10.6	27.5–38.0
6	13.0	14.4–27.4
5	04.9	09.5–14.3
4	04.5	05.0–09.4
3	02.5	02.5–04.9
2	02.0	00.5–02.4
1	00.4	00.0–00.4

Scaled Score Mean = 8.0, Standard Deviation = 2.43

Physical Science

Scaled Score	Percent Achieving Score	Percentile Rank Range
15	00.1	99.9–99.9
14	01.3	98.7–99.9
13	02.1	96.6–98.6
12	04.4	92.2–96.5
11	07.2	85.0–92.1
10	13.9	71.1–84.9
9	11.7	59.4–71.0
8	18.6	40.8–59.3
7	14.0	26.8–40.7
6	13.4	13.4–26.7
5	08.5	04.8–13.3
4	03.4	01.4–04.7
3	01.2	00.3–01.3
2	00.1	00.1–00.2
1	00.0	00.0–00.0

Scaled Score Mean = 8.1, Standard Deviation = 2.32

Writing Sample

Scaled Score	Percent Achieving Score	Percentile Rank Range
T	00.6	99.5–99.9
S	03.2	96.3–99.4
R	09.3	87.0–96.2
Q	12.1	74.9–86.9
P	12.1	62.8–74.8
O	13.1	49.7–62.7
N	12.7	37.1–49.6
M	21.3	15.8–37.0
L	09.5	06.3–15.7
K	04.0	02.3–06.2
J	02.2	00.0–02.2

75th Percentile = Q, 50th Percentile = O, 25th Percentile = M

Biological Sciences

Scaled Score	Percent Achieving Score	Percentile Rank Range
15	00.1	99.9–99.9
14	00.5	99.5–99.8
13	02.4	97.2–99.4
12	04.3	92.9–97.1
11	08.8	84.1–92.8
10	16.0	68.1–84.0
9	15.5	52.6–68.0
8	16.0	36.6–52.5
7	12.6	24.0–36.5
6	09.9	14.1–23.9
5	06.3	07.8–14.0
4	04.6	03.2–07.7
3	02.2	01.0–03.1
2	00.7	00.3–00.9
1	00.2	00.0–00.2

Scaled Score Mean = 8.2, Standard Deviation = 2.39

Prepping for the MCAT

You wouldn't run a marathon without training for it; your chances of doing your best without preparation are practically nil. Similarly, you don't want to go into the MCAT cold. Prepping for the MCAT will help you accomplish three things:

- Learn or review the content on the test
- Build endurance needed to face nearly eight hours of testing
- Gain confidence in your ability to manage the material and the stress of test day

You can prep in a variety of ways, through live courses, software, or books. Kaplan offers thorough preparation for all learning styles and budgets. For more information on the best MCAT prep for you, call 1-800-KAP-TEST.

When to Take It

The MCAT tests your basic knowledge of physics, general chemistry, biology, and organic chemistry. So make sure you take one year of each before taking the MCAT.

The MCAT is offered only twice a year, in April and August. Applications for the MCAT become available in January of

Endurance Testing

The MCAT is a full day of testing, so make sure you are well prepared emotionally and physically. Do a dry run at least once before the real thing.

each year. You should give yourself lots of lead time for getting the information and preparing thoroughly.

Applications for MCAT registration are available from your premed advisor or from the MCAT Program Office:

MCAT Program Office
2255 North Dubuque Road
PO Box 4056
Iowa City, IA 52243
(319) 337-1356

There is no easy answer to the question of whether to take the MCAT in April or August. You will need to decide for yourself based on your own circumstances. There are advantages and disadvantages to both test administrations.

April Advantages:

- The timing is right. Many applicants take the MCAT in the spring of their junior year of college. This is when all of the common prerequisite courses have been completed and these students feel better prepared to take the test.
- Taking the MCAT in April gets it out of the way so you can concentrate on preparing your AMCAS application and other aspects of the application process.
- You will receive your scores in June and this may help you to decide on how many schools to apply to. It may also help you to decide upon particular schools to include on your application list.
- If your scores are below your expectations, you have an opportunity to repeat the test in August.
- You must take the MCAT in April if you wish to apply to your first choice school under the Early Decision Plan.
- Medical schools receive your April scores along with your AMCAS application rather than having to wait until October to receive August scores.
- You may have the support of classmates who are preparing for the MCAT.

April Disadvantages:

- You may not be ready because you have not completed all of the prerequisite courses.
- You may feel that MCAT preparation will take time from your studies and adversely affect your grades.
- Your work schedule may not permit adequate preparation time.

August Advantages:

- You may now have completed all of the prerequisite courses.
- You may have the entire summer to prepare for the test with fewer distractions.
- It may fit into your personal schedule better.

August Disadvantages:

- Your scores will reach the medical schools later in the application season.
- You will not have a chance to repeat the MCAT during the current application year.
- Preparation may limit your other summer options.
- You may not have the support of your classmates who are also preparing for the MCAT.
- Your application file may become complete later in the application year, thus delaying a decision to send supplemental materials to you or to invite you for an interview.
- You will not be able to take advantage of the Early Decision Plan.

How Long Are MCAT Scores Valid?

The current version of the MCAT was introduced in April, 1991. Medical schools that require the MCAT will expect that your scores be no older than that. Some schools have much stricter limits and will only accept scores from more recent test administrations. Consult the individual school entries in the MSAR to determine the oldest MCAT scores they will accept.

Tips for MCAT Success

Here are some tried-and-true strategies for doing your best on the MCAT examination.

- Learn the test components inside and out.
- Consider enrolling in an MCAT prep course.
- Review the content outlined in the MCAT student manual.
- Practice MCAT-style problems in each topic area after you've reviewed the area.
- Build up your test-taking stamina. This is approximately a six-hour test with nearly three extra hours devoted to administrative details and breaks. It's not a good idea to think you can just waltz in and keep alert for all six hours!
- Take all the MCAT practice tests you can. Practice with shorter, focused MCAT practice tests first to increase your accuracy; then tackle longer practice exams to build your testing stamina.

> ### *Take a Guess*
>
> There is no guessing penalty on the MCAT. Never leave a question blank! If you don't know the answer, you can only benefit from guessing.

- Figure out in practice how much time you can spend on each question in each section. Practice moving more quickly so if you fall behind on the test, you've practiced catching up too.
- Learn from your mistakes—get the most out of your practice test experience.
- Learn a step-by-step approach to the writing sample. This is not a freestyle writing test. You will be judged on your ability to communicate clearly and effectively.
- Keep building up your confidence in your test-taking ability. Confidence feeds on itself and results in higher scores.

It's okay to take the MCAT in April of the semester you'll be finishing some of your premed courses.

Health Care Experience

According to a recent survey of medical schools, knowledge of health care issues and commitment to health care were among the top five variables considered very important to student selection (the other four were medical school interview ratings, GPA, MCAT scores, and letters of recommendation). While having experience in health care—most likely some type of volunteer experience—is not exactly a requirement, you should think about being as active in health care activities as possible as a premed student. Consider volunteering in a local hospice, nursing home, or clinic. If nothing else, health care experience will help you articulate in your personal statements and interviews why you want to pursue a career in medicine.

Free Ride

Thirty-four schools currently offer Medical Scientist Training Programs (MSTPs). MSTPs are very competitive M.D.-Ph.D. programs funded by the National Institutes of Health. MSTP students receive tuition allowance and a yearly stipend for up to six years. For more information contact:

Program Administrator
Medical Scientist Training Program
National Institutes of Health
45 Center Drive MSC 6200
Bethesda, MD 20892-6200

(301) 594-3830

Joint Degree Programs

Many medical schools offer joint degree programs, the most common one being the joint M.D./Ph.D. in an area relating to medicine. In 1998–99, 116 schools allowed students to pursue the M.D. and Ph.D. in an area pertinent to medicine, such as biochemistry, immunology, neurosciences, pharmacology, and other related areas. M.D./Ph.D. programs are long—at least six years—and require a high level of commitment.

Some M.D./Ph.D. candidates see the joint degree as a way of achieving balance between clinical medicine and scientific research. Your chance of admission into a joint degree program is based in part on your commitment to both clinical work and research/teaching. If you're considering applying to a joint degree program, make sure you can articulate the reasons why you want to pursue both degrees. The appendix lists the joint degree programs that each med school offers.

CHAPTER 7

Letters of Recommendation

Letters of recommendation are typically submitted with the secondary applications, in the latter part of the application process. However, it's important that you start to think about and solicit your letters much earlier in the game.

Admissions committees are generally very specific about whom they want to submit letters on your behalf. Many committees require letters from either a premed committee, or from senior science professors. Don't take these requirements lightly. You should do everything you can to give the medical schools exactly the kind of letters they have requested; after all, there is a reason they ask for certain recommenders. So the question is, how do you know what kind of letters you will be asked to submit, and how do you go about soliciting these letters?

To learn the type of letters you are likely to be required to send to a particular medical school, visit your premed office. The office should have on file the secondary applications, and therefore the types of letters requested, for every medical school in the country. By taking an early look at the secondary applications of those medical schools to which you are planning to apply, you can get a jump on establishing relationships with the people best suited to write your recommendation letters.

Premedical Committee Letters

It is fairly typical for a medical school to ask you for a "premed committee letter." These letters are typically of two types: either an original letter written by your undergraduate premedical committee on your behalf, or a summary of excerpts of comments made by individuals who have submitted letters (at your request) on your behalf. The premed committee letter used to be a standard component of any applicant's application. Unfortunately, in recent years many institutions have eliminated the premed committee because of cutbacks in funding, which means that many applicants are unable to obtain such a letter. If this is your situation, med schools will accept individual letters in lieu of a committee letter.

Individual Letters

If an applicant is not submitting a premed committee letter, he will typically be asked to submit three individual letters of recommendation. Generally, some if not all of these letters must come from senior science faculty. A letter written by a teaching assistant seldom, if ever, carries as much weight with the admissions committee as does a letter coming from a senior faculty member, and therefore should be avoided if at all possible. However, letters cosigned by both the teaching assistant and professor are generally acceptable. In addition to the recommendations from science faculty, some medical schools request that nonscience majors submit letters from a professor in their major. You may also be asked to submit a letter by someone familiar with your clinical experience.

How to Solicit Letters

If you're like many other applicants, the idea of approaching a professor to ask for a letter of recommendation is chilling. This is particularly true if you are planning to approach a professor whose class you attended years before, or one in which you were one of seven or eight hundred students. The concern, and it is a very real concern, is that letters solicited under these circumstances will be no more than glorified form letters and will be written with very little insight or care.

Your job, therefore, is to put yourself in a position in which your professor(s) get to know you. Notice that we didn't say "put yourself in a position in which you get to know your professors." That misses the point. You're not writing your professor a letter of recommendation; she's writing one for you. So how do you help your professor get to know you? Step one: Start early.

I Like What's-His-Name

Beware the impersonal recommendation. Be sure to ask a potential recommender if he or she can write a strong letter. If not, move on.

While you're completing your premed requirements, visit your professor during office hours if you have any questions regarding course material. Students will often seek out their TA's for assistance, but seldom their professors. Chances are that if you go to see your professor during office hours, you will be one of only a handful of students present. Consider getting a cup of coffee or going to lunch with your professors. Many undergraduate institutions sponsor something called "Take Your Professor to Lunch" to encourage faculty and students to intermingle. What a deal: Not only do you get a free lunch, but you also get to know your professors outside of the classroom. And if you do well in a particular class or have an especially positive experience, apply to become a teaching assistant the following year, or volunteer to work in that professor's lab. The possibilities are limitless; you just need to put forth a little effort to get the relationship started.

When you approach someone to write a letter of recommendation, don't hesitate to ask whether he or she can write you a strong letter of support. If the person hesitates in any way ("I'm going to be out of town"; "I'm really very busy now"; "I don't have any secretarial support"), look elsewhere. While this may be the truth, this may also be a way to tell you that he or she can't, or won't, write a letter on your behalf. Although this may be embarrassing, it will hurt you a lot more in the long run to have someone's late recommendation force you to withdraw your application, or worse yet, to have a lukewarm letter of recommendation submitted.

Assuming the individuals you ask express pleasure and honor at being requested to write a letter on your behalf, be prepared to give them a copy of your résumé to provide a complete picture of your background and interests. If you have a strong academic record, you may want to include a copy of your transcript to showcase your academic prowess and consistency. Any articles or papers that you think may be helpful should also be offered. Finally, always provide recommenders with addressed and stamped envelopes to either your premed advisor/committee or the school in question.

Nontraditional Applicants

Applicants who have been out of undergraduate school for several years face special issues when it comes to obtaining letters of recommendations. Generally speaking, medical schools will still request that you submit letters from undergraduate science professors from whom you took a course. However, it is also likely that you'll be asked to submit letters from employers. Whether you're still in college or long graduated, do everything in your power to provide medical schools with whatever letters they request.

As a nontraditional applicant, you have two options as to how to go about obtaining letters from professors: You can go back to your undergraduate professors, or you can take additional postbaccalaureate science classes at a four-year institution, and ask these professors to write recommendations.

The latter may be the best option for two reasons. First, many medical schools require that prerequisites be done within a certain timeframe; this alone may mean that you'll need to go back to school to take additional courses. Second, depending on the length of time since you last saw your professors, it's possible they're not going to remember you, no matter how sterling your personality.

If you don't have a premed office available to you to coordinate the compilation and sending of your letters, your recommendation writers may send their letters directly to the medical school themselves.

Confidential or Nonconfidential Letters?

When you initially open a file with your premed office, you will be asked to decide whether you want an "open" or "closed" file. Individual medical schools may ask you this question again on their secondary applications. If you choose to have an open file, you will have access to your letters of recommendations. If you do, admissions committees may question whether or not you've "censored" your letters by including in your packet only those that paint a very positive picture of you. Admissions committees want to have assurance that they are receiving a complete, unedited picture of you from those who wrote your letters of evaluation. From the medical schools' perspective, therefore, it is preferable that you have a closed file and that your letters be confidential.

Do the Waive

Conventional wisdom dictates that you should waive your option to review your recommendations. Med schools prefer that you not have any hand in what is written about you in these letters.

What Makes a Great Recommendation?

Keep in mind the purpose of recommendation letters: They serve as outside endorsements of your medical school candidacy. The more personal the letter, the better off you are.

Schools fully expect these letters to be glowing endorsements. Anything less is a red flag. Admissions committees are looking for applicants who have demonstrated intelligence, maturity, integrity, and a dedication to the ideal of service to society—all the things that you'd look for in a physician. To this end, a glowing letter of recommendation generally begins by detailing the circumstances under which the letter writer has come to know the applicant. This includes the length of time and the nature of the association. It then evaluates the candidate on the nature and depth of scholarly and/or extracurricular activities undertaken, the candidate's academic record and performance on MCAT's, the personal and emotional characteristics of the candidate, and finally, the letter writer's overall assessment as to the candidate's suitability for the medical profession. The admissions committee may consider detrimental a letter of recommendation that focuses solely on the academic qualifications of the applicant, and gives little or no attention to the candidate's nonacademic strengths and characteristics.

Timing it All

Don't wait until the fall to ask for letters of recommendation. You don't want to be crushed in the fall rush, when zillions of premeds are scrambling, and science professors are overwhelmed. Waiting until the last minute means that it's likely that the quality of the letters will suffer.

Keep track of the status of your letters. If they're late, call and check on their progress. But don't harass your recommenders; if you make a pest of yourself, it could negatively impact what they will end up writing about you. Once you've confirmed that your letters have been sent, it's nice to send thank-you notes to the writers. Personal visits are in order after you've been accepted.

CHAPTER 8

Submitting Your Application

The medical school application is your single best opportunity to convince a group of strangers that you would be an asset both to the school and the medical profession. It's your opportunity to show yourself as something more than grades and scores. Granted, every person who applies will have strengths and weaknesses. But it's how you present your strengths and weaknesses that counts.

So what's the best way to present yourself on the application? We all know that some people are natural-born sellers in person, but the med school admissions process is written, not spoken. The key here is not natural talent but rather organization—carefully planning a coherent presentation from beginning to end and paying attention to every detail in between.

> ### Develop a Theme
>
> Start thinking early about what theme you want your application to convey. Decide what your real purpose is in applying to medical school, and make sure that this sense of purpose comes through in all aspects of your application.

AMCAS versus Non-AMCAS

AMCAS (American Medical College Application Service) is a centralized application processing service that is based in Washington, D.C. The AMCAS people do not make any admissions decisions. They simply process, duplicate, and send your application and MCAT scores to all AMCAS member schools that you designate, and verify your academic history. The AMCAS application is a godsend—it greatly simplifies the initial stages of the application process. Instead of having to complete individual applications for every single school, you complete just one AMCAS application. All but sixteen of the U.S. LCME-accredited medical schools are AMCAS schools.

You can get an AMCAS application from your premed advisor or career center, or you can contact AMCAS directly:

AMCAS
2501 M Street, NW
Lobby–26
Washington, DC 20037-1300
(202) 828-0600
http://www.aamc.org/stuapps

Schools that don't participate in AMCAS (a.k.a., non-AMCAS schools) have their own, individual applications that you'll need to complete. This must be done for each of the non-AMCAS schools that you apply to, and the applications can differ significantly. Do not send the AMCAS application to a non-AMCAS school; it won't be amused.

AACOMAS

Osteopathic medical schools also maintain a centralized application service called AACOMAS (American Association of Colleges of Osteopathic Medicine Application Service). AACOMAS services all nineteen U.S. osteopathic medical schools, and operates similarly to AMCAS. For more information, contact AACOMAS:

American Association of Colleges of Osteopathic Medicine
5550 Friendship Boulevard
Suite 310
Chevy Chase, MD 20815
(301) 968-4190
http://www.aacom.org

The AMCAS Application

AMCAS applications become available in April for the class entering in the fall of the following year. AMCAS begins accepting applications on June 1. The sooner you obtain the application, the sooner you can complete it; the sooner you can send it in, the better off you'll be. (But don't send it before June 1—it will be returned.) Remember, always try to get a jump on the game. Medical schools will want to see an application form, your transcripts, your MCAT scores, and letters of recommendation before they inform you that your application is complete. Until they receive all the components of your application folder, they will not consider you for a personal interview.

Many schools have instituted a rolling admissions system. This means that those applicants who are reviewed first will be given the first interviews, and subsequently, be granted admission before other candidates. There is seldom a downside for getting your application in as soon after June 1 as possible. Even if you're taking the August MCAT, you should try to get your application in early so medical schools can open a file on you. You'll look eager and organized. That being said, if you can't send it in June or early July, and you find that working on it really cuts into your MCAT prep time—put it away until after the test. You need to focus on getting your best possible MCAT scores, and it isn't detrimental to get the AMCAS application in later (but no later than September), since schools won't consider your application until they have your August MCAT scores anyway.

> **Get the Worm**
>
> Does it really pay to go to a lot of trouble to apply early? Yes, particularly in the era of rolling admissions. If you delay and submit your applications late in the season, schools may have no openings left.

Although some schools don't employ rolling admissions, they nonetheless begin assessing applications as soon as they are received, and consequently, will begin to offer interviews to those who they feel are qualified candidates. This is a major advantage: If you send your materials in too late, you will be given an interview later in the application season. Some schools will discuss candidates they have met and discussed at the last admissions committee meeting at subsequent meetings. So, if you've interviewed in October, you could be reviewed five times; if you interview in March, you've got one shot. Again, the moral of the story is to be prepared. Do not procrastinate.

AMCAS Application Details

The AMCAS application consists of three sections:

1. General information (Education, Work, Activities, Honors)
2. Personal statement
3. Coursework and GPA calculations

General Information

The information requested is similar to what you find in almost any kind of application. Avoid the "throw everything in and the kitchen sink" mentality. You want to spotlight those activities and honors that are most important to you and the ones that you hope will distinguish your application. Always list in order of decreasing priority. You may also want to highlight health-related activities, public service work, and science or medically related research experience. Common sense will serve you well here.

> **Follow Directions**
>
> Admissions officers are amazed at how many applicants simply refuse to follow directions. Don't think that you're an exception to any rule. If the application asks for X, give them X, not Y.

Personal Statement

The personal statement is such a crucial—and anxiety producing—part of the application that we've devoted an entire chapter to it. See chapter 9 for detailed information.

Coursework and GPA Calculations

The AMCAS application requires that you input a detailed list of just about every course you've taken since secondary school. Before you even begin, you should have a copy of an unofficial transcript from all undergrad and grad institutions you've attended. You'll need this to tackle the complex matrix of classes, semester hours, credits, and grades.

Apply Electronically

The AMCAS electronic application is called AMCAS-E, while AACOMAS calls it the AACOMAS Computerized Application. You can complete you application on computer and submit your data on disk to the appropriate application service. Paper applications are also accepted by both organizations.

If you're using AMCAS-E, the software will convert your grades to AMCAS's scale. If you're using the paper version, it's a bit more complex. After you've accounted for all your courses and grades, you'll need to refer to the Grading Systems Conversion Table in your AMCAS instruction booklet so that you can convert your grades to AMCAS's scale. You should also complete the AMCAS GPA Calculation Sheet so you aren't surprised to learn how AMCAS arrived at your GPA.

The AMCAS-E and AACOMAS computerized applications mean that you won't have to struggle with printing information in tiny boxes; you'll be able to fill out your application on computer and submit your disk to the application service. Whether you're working on paper or disk, check and double-check your work.

When you complete and mail your AMCAS application, you'll be required to have official transcripts forwarded to AMCAS from every school you've attended after high school. Generally, colleges charge for this service. For each school you've attended, call ahead to find out its particular procedures and charges for sending transcripts.

Transcript Requests

AMCAS-E includes transcript requests on the disk. If you're using the paper form, request transcripts with the transcript matching cards enclosed in the AMCAS booklet. Though using the card is not required, it can help you avoid confusion. With any correspondence you have with AMCAS, always include your full name, official address, and social security number.

Application Dos and Don'ts

Don't Use Application Forms or Disks from Previous Years.
Most applications change from year to year.

Always Double- and Triple-Check Your Application for Spelling Errors.
You lose a certain amount of credibility if you write that you were a "Roads Scholar."

Check for Accidental Contradictions.
Make sure that your application doesn't say you worked in a hospital in 1995 when your financial aid forms say you were driving a cab that year.

Prioritize All Lists.
When a question asks you to list your honors or awards, don't begin with fraternity social chairman and end with Phi Beta Kappa. Let the admissions committee know that you realize what's important—always list significant scholastic accomplishments first.

Account for All of Your Time.
If you have been away from school for longer than a semester, did not enter college directly from high school, have been out of college for some time, or had other breaks in your education, be sure that your application shows what you were doing during that period. Don't leave gaps.

Don't Overdo Listing Extracurricular Activities.
Don't list every event or every activity you ever participated in. Select the most significant and, if necessary, explain them. Admissions officers are suspicious of people who list twenty-five time-consuming extracurricular activities and yet still manage to attend college.

Don't Mention High School Activities or Honors.
Unless there's something very unusual or spectacular about your high school background, don't mention it. Yes, this means not taking note of the fact that you were senior class president. However, you should list health-related work or volunteering.

Juggling Act

When juggling several applications at once, it's easy to make careless mistakes. Double-check yourself at every step.

Clear Up Any Ambiguities.

On questions concerning employment, for instance, make sure to specify whether you held a job during the school year or only during the summer. Many applications ask about this, and it may be an important point to the admissions officer.

Lone Star

The state of Texas has its own application form for state schools. To apply to the UT system, write:

Application Service
Texas Medical and Dental Schools
Suite 6.400, 702 Colorado
Austin, TX 78701
Tel: (512) 499-4785
http://dpweb1.dp.utexas.edu/mdac/

Non-AMCAS Applications

Not surprisingly, most of the non-AMCAS schools provide applications similar in content to the AMCAS application. These applications also contain general information pages, and of course, an essay (one or more). The major difference may be that a non-AMCAS school simply requests a copy of your transcript, rather than making you compute yearly and subject GPAs, as is the case with the AMCAS application. Since there is so much overlap, once you have completed the AMCAS application, you shouldn't have much difficulty cranking out the non-AMCAS applications. You probably can take most of your personal statement from the AMCAS application.

Non-AMCAS Schools

For 2001, the following will need to be contacted individually for applications (schools not listed participated in the AMCAS program):

- Baylor College of Medicine
- Brown University School of Medicine
- Canadian Schools of Medicine (16 schools)
- Columbia University College of Physicians and Surgeons
- New York University School of Medicine
- Texas A&M University School of Medicine
- Texas Tech University Health Sciences Center School of Medicine
- University of North Dakota School of Medicine
- University of Missouri—Kansas City School of Medicine
- University of Texas System (Southwestern, Galveston, Houston, and San Antonio)

Secondaries

So you finally finish your AMCAS and/or non-AMCAS applications. You relax and congratulate yourself on completing all that darned paperwork. You put away the checkbook and sit back to await your interview invitations. Well, don't get too comfy, because there is more paperwork on the way! Nearly all schools will forward a secondary application after they receive your AMCAS or non-AMCAS applications. As noted earlier, some schools will send secondaries to all applicants, while others will screen their candidate pools before sending secondaries. What do the secondaries entail? Well, they can vary from demanding just a little more biographical information, to requesting full-fledged essays. The one thing they almost uniformly request: more money (surprise, surprise). It's usually at the secondary application stage that you'll be asked to forward your letters of recommendation. Again, in secondaries you explain your interest in individual schools, so do your research.

Managing Your Campaign

When you submit the various components of your application is as important as *what* you submit: If you miss deadlines or don't remember to include a piece of necessary information, your stellar GPA and MCAT scores, brilliant personal statement, or glowing recommendations are for naught. The moral: Keep yourself organized.

No Seconds

For the 2000 entering class, the following schools did not require an additional secondary application fee:

- Medical College of Georgia
- Uniformed Services U. of Health Sciences
- U. of Arizona
- U. of Mississippi
- U. of Texas schools

CHAPTER 9

The Personal Statement

When you submit an AMCAS application, you have the opportunity to "talk" to the admissions committee members via your one-page "Personal Comments." You may use this space to write about anything you want. Applicants often wonder whether their statement is actually read by the admissions committee. Not only will it be read, it will be read again and again during the application process.

While your academic history is a reflection of your potential to successfully negotiate the medical school curriculum, your personal statement is the first step in developing a portrait of who you are as a person and whether or not you have the personality traits and characteristics necessary to be a physician.

While it is impossible to know what each medical school is looking for when it reviews your personal statement, it is nonetheless the one area in which you can infuse a little bit of personality. As with all creative outlets, there is no single correct way to go about this, no simple formula to follow. Your goal in writing your statement should be to make yourself a "real person" to the admissions committee and not just an "academic profile." Using your life story to illustrate the points you are trying to make is an excellent way of doing this.

What to Write

When applicants write their personal statements, they often try so hard to sound impressive to the admissions committee that their writing style becomes stilted and artificial. These applicants wind up portraying themselves as overstuffed, pompous characters no committee member would want to spend much time with, instead of providing accurate portraits of themselves.

Here are some important points to consider, as well as common pitfalls to avoid when writing your statement.

- The personal statement is not the time to recount all your activities and honors in listlike fashion. Avoid writing the rehashed résumé or typical biographical essay ("I was born in a small fishing village . . .").

> ### *Weave a Story*
>
> Use vignettes and anecdotes to make your essay a pleasure to read. Why did you decide to go into medicine? Was it an experience you had in school? Have you or family members had an experience with the medical community that left a lasting impression? Be creative.

- Make it personal. This is your opportunity to put a little panache into the application. Show the admissions committee why you decided to go into medicine.
- Be yourself. This is not the time to try on a new persona, nor is it the time to fall back on clichés. Unless you're one of the five people in the world who is naturally funny, it is probably not a good idea to start your personal statement with a joke.
- Don't name drop; no one will be impressed.
- Don't write in the third person. Normal people do not write about themselves as though they were writing about someone else.
- Don't begin every sentence with the pronoun *I*, since doing so makes you sound egotistical.

- You probably want to avoid delving into any controversial topics, such as abortion or euthanasia. If you do decide to include one, though, definitely avoid being dogmatic or preachy. You don't want to take the risk of alienating a reader who may not share your politics.
- Try not to make apologies for your past. For instance, if you received a C in physics (hey, it could happen), don't feel compelled to justify it somehow. However, there may be events in your past for which you believe the circumstances truly do merit some mention. When this is the case, briefly state the relevant facts, but don't make excuses. What you don't want to do is provide the admissions committee with a road map to your weakness by making the problem bigger than it really is. On the other hand, if there really is a weakness in your application, avoiding the issue will not prevent the admissions committee from finding it on its own. If you haven't provided a context in which to view the issue, you may not have an opportunity to do so again. If further information is needed, your premed adviser will be able to explain details in his or her cover letter.
- You can't take liberties with margins or fonts with AMCAS-E, since margins will be preset and fonts will be standardized. That means that you'll have to write a personal statement of the appropriate length—no rambling on for pages, or trying to turn a paragraph into a page. If you're submitting a paper application, stay with preset borders and type in a font no smaller than a point size of 12.

The Five Most Common Mistakes

We asked a medical school admissions officer for the five most common mistakes students make in writing their personal statements. Here's what she told us:

Underestimating the Importance of the Essay

It appears to be a common misperception that a stellar academic record will overcome other deficiencies in a student's application, including a poorly written personal statement. This is often glaringly evident when a student writes a few hastily constructed paragraphs, leaving most of the allotted page blank. In other less obvious examples, it is apparent that students simply haven't allotted enough time to work through several drafts of the essay to arrive at a solidly constructed personal statement.

Using Excessive Detail—the "Overwhelm and Conquer" Approach

This common misperception—that more is better—results in an essay that generates groans from the unfortunate reader on the admissions committee. The student who gives credence to this approach is forced to use a barely readable type size to fill every inch of the allotted page. Unfortunately, it is such an unpleasant experience for the reader to wade through this essay that the entire application often goes to the bottom of the pile.

Failing to Make the Essay Personal

A very common mistake is to use the essay to recite a list of activities and accomplishments, without really addressing the question, "Why medicine?" When students fail to convey what they actually learned from their experiences, they fail to communicate to an admissions committee how they see themselves as an asset to both the medical school and the medical profession.

Embellishing the Essay

Students often avoid the personal approach entirely by writing an overly creative or philosophical treatise, hoping to impress the committee with their unique approach. While this approach may be interesting reading, it does not leave the reader with a compelling reason to recommend the student for an interview. There is a place for creativity in the essay, but overall, the personal statement should not deviate from the standard essay format.

Failing to Proofread the Essay

Attention to detail often eludes the medical school applicant. The failure to proofread can be a devastating omission, as nothing destroys the credibility of an application faster than misspelled words and faulty grammar. Admissions committees place a high value on strong communication skills—both written and verbal—and expect high quality writing in the personal statement.

Writing Drafts

Because the personal statement is such an important part of your application, it shouldn't be done overnight. A strong personal statement may take shape over the course of weeks or months and will require several different drafts. Write a draft and then let it sit for a few weeks. Time gives you valuable perspective on something you've written. If you leave it alone for a significant period of time you may find (to your astonishment) that your first instincts were good ones; on the other hand, you may shudder at how you could ever have considered submitting such a piece of garbage.

Allow at least a month or so to write your statement, and don't be afraid to overhaul it completely if you're not satisfied. Most important, get several different perspectives. Have close friends or relatives read it to see if it really captures what you want to convey, asking them about their initial reactions as well as their feelings after studying it more carefully. Once you've achieved a draft that you feel comfortable with, try to have it read by a few people who barely know you or by people who don't know you at all. Such people may include professors unfamiliar with your work, college advisers other than your own, or friends of friends. Strangers or semistrangers often provide a better perspective on your work than those close to you. Since they haven't heard the story before and don't know the characters, they're often better able to tell you when something is missing or confusing.

Proofread!

Proofreading is of critical importance. Don't be afraid to enlist the aid of others. If possible, let an English teacher review the essay solely for spelling and grammar mistakes. Nothing catches an admissions officer's eye more quickly than a misspelled word.

The bottom line is to let a reasonable number of people read the essay and make suggestions. To avoid being overly influenced by an individual reader, try to read all of the comments at once. If certain criticisms are consistently made, then they're probably legitimate. But don't be carried away by every suggestion every reader makes. Stick to your basic instincts—after all, this is your personal statement, not someone else's.

The Interview Connection

Interviewers often use your personal statement as fodder for questions. They may focus on a couple of key points mentioned in your essay and use these as springboards for discussion. If you have included experiences and ideas that are dear to you or that you feel strongly about, you will have no problem speaking with passion and confidence. Nothing is more appealing to admissions folks than a vibrant, intelligent, and articulate candidate. If you write about research you conducted five years ago, you'd better brush up before your interviews. Think about the following:

- What was the purpose of your research? Was it part of a larger research question?
- What benefit came out of your research?
- Is there a relevant history to your research?

- What exactly did you do?
- Whether or not your research was ultimately successful, what did you learn?

While letters of recommendations serve as outside endorsements, the personal statement is your own personal sales pitch. You're up against thousands and thousands of qualified candidates. You have to make yourself stand out from the crowd. Everyone has a story to tell. The key lies in how you tell your own tale.

Institutional Action

Admissions committees are very concerned with the moral character of potential physicians. Because of this, the AMCAS application asks whether you've ever been the subject of an institutional action. This question must be answered truthfully and completely in the "personal comments" section of the application. In addition, you may be asked to provide documentation or discuss the incident further in an interview.

Because an institutional action—particularly one resulting from a conduct violation—may say something about a candidate's integrity, medical school admissions committees view it very seriously. However, an institutional action will not necessarily prevent admission. Each situation is considered individually in the context of mitigating factors leading up to and surrounding the incident, insight shown by the applicant into his or her behavior, and the candidate's perspective on the incident in retrospect.

Real Essays, Real Responses

Below are three essays that were submitted by three students applying to medical school last year. Following each essay are the comments of two admissions officers from two different medical schools, each of whom were given the essays to critique without the rest of the students' applications. As you read the comments, notice that while each of the admissions officers seems to have an individual slant on what he or she thinks are the positive and negative points of each essay, they agree on the larger points: that essays should be personal, well written, convincing, and should clearly answer the question, "why medicine?"

Essay One

Robert F. Kennedy, during a campaign speech for the Presidency of the United States, said that "Tragedy is a tool for the living to gain wisdom, not a guide by which to live." It was a Friday night, on August 28th, 1992, when I was compelled to live that quotation. On the way home from Sabbath services with my parents, two sisters, and brother, our car was struck by a drunk driver, killing my sister Sarah and severely injuring my family. As I lay in the hospital bed, tubes and machines surrounding me, I could only foresee a life of despondency.

Now, five years later, I understand Kennedy's words; my despondency has changed into a strong commitment to help others. Less than a year after the accident, I took a course to become a certified emergency medical technician (EMT), having learned from first-hand experience the importance of basic life-saving skills, I was determined to gain that knowledge. Once in college, I became actively involved with the Brandeis Emergency Medical Corps (BEMCo), an organization of volunteer EMTs who respond to all emergency medical calls on campus.

The summer between my freshman and sophomore year, I worked for a private ambulance service in Los Angeles. I found this experience very valuable because it brought me into the inner-city for the first time. I was exposed to individuals who lived on a daily basis with fear and uncertainty about their health when some of the finest medical technology was just moments away. Intrigued by these issues, I later enrolled in a specialized health, law and medicine program at Brandeis to study possible solutions to the problems I saw.

By the end of my sophomore year, I knew that I wanted to see for myself and learn more about the effects of diseases on the body. As a result, I took an internship at the UCLA Department of Pathology, where I began assisting in autopsies. I was able to apply the textbook description and organ functions that I had previously learned into their clinical aspects. From this experience, I not only acquired a greater appreciation of how the human body functions, but I also learned that bodies are more than just organs and series of chemical reactions.

I have come to realize that there is no deeper way of understanding the human face of medicine than to be a patient or clinician oneself. When I was growing up in France, my family and I had built a deep-rooted relationship with our family physician. Dr. Celan knew each of our personal and medical history, and with love, attention, confidence, and trust cared for us and his other patients. I know from the accident that being alone in an emergency room can be very frightening. I also know that regardless of how may shots of anesthetics I received that night, nothing helped me more and gave me more strength than holding my doctor's hand. A simple human approach can bring significant results.

While no activity I take part in will ever bring my sister back, I can and will forever strive for the strength to take what I have learned from the accident and help others in her memory. I am now starting my fourth year in BEMCo. I have the primary responsibility for our three-person team, and I am one of two supervisors for the Corps. Every time that I respond to an emergency, I look at the patient and see Sarah's beautiful face. I am reminded each time that even if I do not know these patients, they are still as important to someone as Sarah was and is to my family.

Comments of Admissions Officer One

Admissions committees rely on the student's essay in the personal statement as one tool to assess the personal qualities that are deemed significant in future medical students and physicians. They seek mature, intelligent, and compassionate individuals who are also positive, articulate, and goal-directed—in essence, individuals who will excel in the art of medicine, as well as the science of medicine. Essays are examined with an eye to how successfully the student has achieved the goal of communicating to an admissions committee that he or she will be an asset both to the medical school and the medical profession.

This essay is a pleasure to critique as it embodies the elements that craft a successful personal statement. The student draws upon a compelling personal experience, along with a powerful quotation, to develop the thematic thread that unifies the essay. The introductory section of the essay immediately piques the interest of the reader with its clarity and articulation of purpose. The student's assertion of a "strong commitment to help others" is not merely the words often quoted by premedical students when asked "Why medicine?" This student is able to describe a variety of medically related experiences that support and give credence to his motivation to pursue a medical career. The essay explores the student's logical progression of decisions in his quest to gain an in-depth knowledge of the medical profession. His choice of academic study reflects an individual who is motivated to understand the deeper issues of health care and serve as a problem solver.

This well-crafted essay succeeds in presenting the strength of the candidate's personal qualities—his maturity, confidence, intelligence, and compassion. The student presents himself as a winner—someone who stands out from the crowd—and his originality flows naturally through this essay. Given that other factors in the application are competitive, it is likely that an admissions committee would view this student as a potentially strong candidate both for its medical school and the medical profession.

Comments of Admissions Officer Two

A quick reading of this personal statement leaves this reviewer with an excellent impression of the applicant, who appears to be the type of person that you would enjoy interviewing for medical school. The essay is above average in quality; it captures the reader's attention immediately through the description of a personal tragedy and continues with a chronological outline of extracurricular activities to test the applicant's motivation for medicine.

A closer examination of the personal statement indicates that it is written in classical essay style and presents a number of interesting topics that would form the basis of a meaningful discussion with an interviewer. The first paragraph outlines the genesis of the motivation for medicine as a result of the tragic loss of a sister. In the second paragraph, the applicant's motivation for medicine is clearly stated along with a strong statement of social commitment to help people. This is exactly what the experienced admissions committee member is looking for in a future physician, and precisely what the present-day changing world of medicine needs. Furthermore, the applicant took the initiative to take an EMT course and participate in emergency medical calls, and thereby has tested his motivation through a hands-on situation.

More hands-on experience and a learning experience about other cultures makes the third paragraph a powerful statement. The words express a social consciousness and a concern for people of other cultures that are less fortunate than the applicant—traits that would put the applicant in good standing with the admissions committee. Enrolling in the health, law, and medicine program indicates just how motivated the applicant was to learn about the health-care system.

The fourth and fifth paragraphs present an interesting literary and medical contrast that is rather effective. The applicant has expanded his experience and commented in a cogent manner on two contrasting medical specialties, pathology and family medicine. He demonstrates considerable insight when he comments on the value of "holding (his) doctor's hand." A role model, Dr. Celan, has been identified by the applicant, suggesting that he appreciates that physician's humane characteristics and would administer to patients in a similar fashion.

The final paragraph completes the literary theme and returns to thoughts of the deceased sibling and reinforces the reason for this applicant's deep motivation for medicine. Mentioning that this is his fourth year as an EMT at school, and that he has prime responsibility for a team, will be noted by an admissions committee. This suggests the presence of several attributes that interviewers look for in applicants: a sense of accomplishment, a commitment to service, and leadership qualities.

This reviewer's summary impression is that this personal statement is above average in quality because the pertinent information is presented with a well-connected motivational theme. One gets the impression that the applicant possesses desirable characteristics for the practice of medicine. The person described is mature, motivated to practice medicine, thoughtful, energetic, people-oriented, and understands the human condition.

Essay Two

Last Sunday as I came back from the church buses for the children's ministry, one man asked how it went and I said good. He then commented, "Well, it's different every week. I've been here seven years and it's different every week," which caused me to smile. How fortunate that it is different every week. There will never be a loss of finding something to do, or someone new to meet and listen to.

When volunteering at Cancer Treatment Center on Mondays, I expect the patient visits will be good . . . but I never really know. I do not know if the patient that spoke to me for thirty minutes last week about her daughter will even be conscious enough to recognize my face that day. I do not know if I will encounter hope, hostility, or sadness. I remember one morning I walked into a dim room where a bearded man sat looking into the distance, though looking at a wall. His eyes were somber and completely lost in the knowledge of his condition. He began to ramble about the news his doctor had given him—that he should go home and set his life in order before the cancer totally took him over. He muttered about this place being his last hope and now he would have to fly home that day. As I left the center, I informed my supervisor of the situation and suggested that a chaplain be sent to this man's room. That morning I was brought to face the limitations of medicine, and was glad to discern it from a handicap. Medicine is not a perfect field with the solutions to save the world, but a piece of service to mankind. It addresses those who have hope for physical well-being as well as those who do not.

I find I cannot go back to my high school days when my dreams of being a doctor simulated visions of a clean, tidy office full of cute babies waiting to be examined. Several years ago I spent a summer shadowing my father during his ENT surgeries. It was my pride that kept me concentrating on standing up straight and breathing deep as the sterile surgical smell filled my nostrils and tempted me to collapse at the sight of tonsils scooped out like ice cream. It has been these types of experiences that have injected a shot of realism into my dreams and thus changed my perceptions of how it will be in the lush fields of medicine and how I fit in. I will work with people who have problems entirely real and more threatening than my trivial worries have ever been. These people will be of all ages, professions, and levels of society. They will also need someone in whom to entrust their health—their security. I meet these people every day, and they have no clue that I notice or would like to help. I see the redheaded man who develops my film at the one hour photo has a limp, and wonder if it is a recurring injury or from a recent accident. My hairdresser says she will give birth in just a month and I sit secretly wishing to be there and assist in the miracle. My father begins recovery free from a long month of radiation treatment, and I can only pray and hope to love him enough.

I have asked myself again and again if being a physician is really who I am, or if there is something else. After wrestling with this question, I realized that being a physician is not who I am, though it is an integral part of me. Growing up under the shadow of my father, his example has shaped my ideology to believe that being an instrument in restoring others to health actually changes lives—and this is what I have grown to be a part of and is irrevocably a part of me. It is through this connection with medicine that I see my paradigms of the world shift, and wake up to find that each day is different, new, and challenging.

Comments of Admissions Officer One

It is evident that the student did not place a high priority on writing this essay for his personal statement. The essay suffers from several deficiencies; the most obvious is the lack of an organizing theme. A strong statement of purpose in the opening paragraph is essential to give the reader a sense of direction as the essay unfolds. Unfortunately, the student's thoughts are vague and rambling and it is difficult to understand what the student is trying to say. (What is meant when he states that medicine is "a piece of service to mankind" in paragraph two?) The student's language reflects a lack of sophistication that reflects a serious weakness in his written communication skills. The reader can only conclude that the essay was hastily written and without consultation to improve its structure and content.

While the essay lacks strength and cohesiveness, it speaks volumes as to the state of mind of the writer. The student's writing lacks energy, enthusiasm, and self-confidence. His view of medicine is immature and without adequate grounding in reality. In fact, his reference to "growing up under the shadow of my father" leaves the reader with serious concerns about the student's actual motivation to pursue medicine as a career. Is this his decision, or his father's? It appears that the student's view of medicine has been adopted, rather than acquired. The student has failed to answer the critical question "Why medicine?" in a way that relates to him, personally. The issue of how to revise this essay is moot in comparison to the larger issue: The student needs to come out from under his father's shadow to mature and develop his own identity. When that is accomplished, he will be able to clearly articulate his motivation for a medical career and convince an admissions committee that he will be an asset to the profession.

Comments of Admissions Officer Two

A first read of this personal statement left this reviewer with the impression that the various thoughts, some of which are very good, are not well connected because of an awkward style of composition and poor wording. Nevertheless, this applicant from a physician's household demonstrates a nurturing quality complemented by a social commitment, and may warrant additional review by an admissions committee.

The first paragraph is poorly composed and detracts from the start of the personal statement. This reviewer's guess is that the writer was attempting to demonstrate that she likes working with children at church, and that meeting and talking with people is a natural inclination. These are necessary qualities for a future primary-care physician.

The second paragraph would have made a better opening statement because it demonstrates a testing of the applicant's motivation for medicine and some important personal characteristics for the practice of medicine. Volunteering at the cancer center demonstrates the applicant's motivation and provides "reality testing." The effective part of this paragraph is the applicant's reaction to the depressed moribund patient. This is the highlight of the essay. The applicant's recognizing the symptoms, informing the supervisor, and suggesting a course of action is what medicine is all about. These actions suggest that the writer is a sensitive, mature, take-charge, and nurturing individual.

The third paragraph loses its intended impact because of the fragmented writing style. A rewrite or expansion into the major portion of the essay would serve to greatly enhance the impact of the personal statement. However, the paragraph as written conveys a meaningful message. To this reviewer, several attractive traits are conveyed: a long-standing interest in medicine; a realistic view of the field, gained by observing surgical procedures and volunteering; willingness to be a physician to a wide spectrum of society; and an interest in the human condition.

The poor writing at the essay's end diminishes the impact of what could be a revealing, introspective statement. The writer seems to be unclear as to whether she is self-motivated to pursue a medical career, or is just following her father's desires. This is a legitimate question for any child of a physician, and it demonstrates maturity, independence, and a reasonable level of introspection. To the applicant's credit, the essay ends with an expression of optimism for the future and a spirit of adventure.

This reviewer's final judgment of this personal statement places it in the below-average range because the desultory composition and rudimentary syntax detract too greatly from the considerable substance that the candidate may have. The apparent first-draft quality of the statement may place the candidate in jeopardy of being overlooked—as you write, so shall you be judged.

Essay Three

The most vivid image I have from this past year is that of a twelve year-old child running up and throwing her arms around her pediatrician and giving him a hug hello. Clinically, Violet was wasted, immunilogically depressed, and had the height of an eight year-old and the weight of a six year-old. The sores in her mouth prevented her from eating normally; she fed herself through a valve known as a "PEG tube" that poked out just northeast of her belly-button. But now, in the presence of her doctor, she was glowing.

She didn't get along terribly well with her classmates when she was well enough to go to school. Word got out that she was HIV+ and the kids around her taunted her about it until she cried. Her mother wasn't any better. She ignored Violet on her good days, beat her on the bad ones. She told me that she would feed her daughter dog food when she didn't feel like cooking. It seemed as if a dark cloud enveloped Violet when her mother would enter the room. But as soon as Dr. K walked in, that cloud lifted away and was replaced by a sparkling smile that widened her emaciated face. He was her friend.

During the course of my studies at the Tulane University School of Public Health and Tropical Medicine I saw a lot of patients like Violet. Some sicker, some healthier. Some older, some younger. Some richer, some poorer. I studied their charts and, more importantly, I studied them. Whether I was at their bedside in the hospital, at the busy clinic just a stones-throw away from the housing projects, or in a consultation office somewhere in the rural bayous of Louisiana, I learned to listen to patients and absorb what I saw and what they felt. The volumes of charts I examined for my research filled out the blanks in my spreadsheets. My coursework in biostatistics and epidemiology enabled me to analyze the data and look for trends. The numbers told me that, yes, pediatric AIDS patients' nutritional status does improve with aggressive nutritional support and drug therapy despite the fact that there is no uniformly successful treatment for cryptosporidiosis. This research will likely be published. But while my charts and graphs deftly illustrate quantity of life, talking to a patient face to face provoked thoughts about quality of life. I started to think about which was more important: a patient's serum albumin level or his desire to get out of the darn hospital so he can get home and play ball with the neighborhood kids. I didn't come up with any answers, just more questions.

After our visit with Violet, Dr. K told me that a smile like hers made him forget about all of the bad things that he'd seen that day, if only for a moment. I believe that the reverse is also true: For a moment, Violet forgot that she was dying. She found comfort in the presence of her doctor. The high quality of care that she received came not only from the years of training that her physician completed, but also from the person who dedicated his life to making his patients feel well in every sense of the word.

Comments of Admissions Officer One

The writer of this essay succeeds in weaving a compelling story with compassion and sensitivity. The story of "Violet" creates the thematic thread that unifies this student's essay. Within that thematic context, the student presents important details of her own experiences in both the medical and research arenas. These experiences reveal a depth of understanding of the strengths as well as the limitations of medicine, from first-hand experience with the rich and the poor. Her writing style is simple and direct, with an eloquence that speaks to her depth of understanding. The student's statement, "I learned to listen to patients and absorb what I saw and what they felt" (paragraph three) is supported by the insightful manner in which she writes.

How well does this essay communicate the student's desirability as a candidate to medical school? Clearly, this student possesses many of the personal qualities that admissions committees are seeking in candidates—such as maturity, compassion, and intelligence. She has the ability to communicate in a direct and articulate manner, and demonstrates a realistic understanding of the medical field from both the clinical and research arenas. What is problematic in this essay is that the student fails to make a direct statement as to motivation—why does she want to be a doctor? The conclusion of the essay begs for an articulation of the student's personal goals and ambitions for her own place in medicine. It is a major omission in an otherwise well-written essay. One of the pitfalls of using another person's story as the focus of an essay is that the writer often becomes secondary to the story. If her essay is to succeed with an admissions committee, it is critical for the student to understand that she needs to answer the question "Why medicine?" in a personal way.

Comments of Admissions Officer Two

A quick reading yields a first impression of a well-written essay with poignantly described patient situations and very perceptive descriptions of the attending physicians. One gains the impression that this individual is either a re-applicant, or recently motivated to apply to medical school while in a graduate public health program. In either case, an explanation of the applicant's motivation for wanting to be a physician would greatly enhance her chances for being considered a highly desirable candidate.

The first paragraph is a splendid way to begin a personal statement in a medical school application, since it will likely evoke a favorable response from every pediatrician sitting on the admissions committee. The humanistic facets of the statement could be elaborated on with considerable advantage. The writer seems to be highly observant of the condition of the young AIDS patient, as well as of human behavior—good traits for anyone entering medicine. The only detractor is the misspelling of "immunologically"; a graduate student working in this area of research should not make that mistake.

The second paragraph lacks a description of the writer's personal involvement, but the descriptive narrative is touching and indicates that sensitivity as an observer. The lengthy third paragraph, in which the writer describes her research, is nicely written and presents the fact that she has experienced patient interactions in various clinical settings. It also manifests a personal interest in the patients, but this leads to more introspection. The writer missed a golden opportunity to clearly state that she wants to be a physician so that she can help people like those described. One thinks that perhaps the writer may not want to be a practicing physician, but would rather continue in the field of epidemiology.

The final paragraph is well written and follows the pattern of a classic essay by returning to the opening statement and presenting some cogent observations. The comments indicate that the writer is a sensitive individual who has gained considerable insight about the doctor-patient relationship. This would have been the ideal place to clearly state her desire to be a physician like the one described.

In summary, the writer of this well-written essay has selected a terrific topic and demonstrated insight, yet remains for the most part a reporter of the human drama observed. Since the writer fails to declare an interest in medicine, or to even state a desire to help people, the narrative's impact is lessened. The writer had several opportunities to express her goals; had this been done, the essay would have been above average in quality and certainly would have had an excellent impact on an admissions committee. In the absence of clearly stated goals in the health sciences, the writer may be at a disadvantage in the admissions process of the more clinically oriented schools.

In Summary

The personal statement gives you an invaluable opportunity to describe who you are and why you want to be a physician. Use it to your advantage: Start thinking well in advance about what you want to say to the medical schools to which you are applying, and make sure you put great care into drafting and honing your essay so that it clearly illuminates your individuality as well as your desire to enter the field of medicine.

CHAPTER 10

The Interview

The final step in the evaluation process involves a personal interview. The medical profession is the only profession that requires a personal interview for entry. This fact alone should provide a powerful statement as to the importance admissions committees place on your performance at the interview.

There is a fair amount of mythology surrounding the medical school interview. Much of this stems from the legacy of the "stress interview." One of our favorite tales is this classic passed from one generation of premeds to the next: The interviewer asks the unsuspecting candidate to open a window. As hard as he tries, he can't open it. Why? Because it's nailed shut. (We believe that this story is apocryphal.)

You can rest assured that stress interviews are the rare exception, not the rule. But the interview is an assessment of your composure and maturity. You may be asked a question that makes you uneasy. If something weird or stressful does happen, keep your cool. (For example, if the window incident happened to you, a good response would be, "It appears to be stuck." An inappropriate reaction would be to throw a tantrum or a chair.)

The Interview and Admissions

Since medical schools are inundated with applications, most admissions committees use the interview as the means for making the final selection. Whereas the first round in the admissions process—reviewing your numbers—may seem impersonal, the interview introduces an element of humanity. Here is where you can let your personality and charm really shine through.

Once you have reached the interview stage, the academic differences among applicants become more subtle. Committees look for trends or patterns of behavior as a means of distinguishing one applicant from the next. They will look at exactly what courses you took to get those A's, and they'll ask themselves the following questions:

- Were there any community colleges listed in the official transcript? Why?
- Did you achieve competency in a foreign language? (Studying medical school vocabulary and information requires many of the same skills that learning a language demands.)
- Did you take advanced-level courses, or easier ones?
- Did you use AP credits to place out of a subject, or to place you into a higher level?
- How many pass-fail classes have you taken? Were these required or elective courses?
- Do you have a pattern of withdrawing from classes?

The interview means the school thinks you can do the academic work, and that you have something else to offer. As one dean put it, "Brilliance in a doctor doesn't hurt, but we know there are many other attributes that it takes to get through medical school. Persistence, balance, determination: These things are important too."

Individual School Needs

A school will often have an unwritten "flavor" that the committee tries to build. For example, a committee might always tend to favor "niceness" in a class, but might attempt in a particular year to accept more students interested in surgery or primary care. Or, it might look for students with a more geographic or minority representation.

Talk to medical students who attended your undergraduate school to find out if a school tends to favor a unique quality. You can find out who they are from your premed advisor. Call the medical school's office of student education or student affairs to get the students' addresses. Some schools will not release phone numbers, but many will. Don't try to figure this out on the day of the interview, however; you'll have enough to think about.

Bone Up

It's a good idea to keep a copy of your secondary application with your catalog, so you can review them both the night before your interview.

The Interview Day

Most medical school interviews start with an introduction, followed by a tour, after which come two interviews. That means that half of the day is dedicated to a tour of the facilities, and half to two half-hour to 45-minute interviews. Schools will tend to schedule between three and twenty students per day, most around twelve to fifteen. Expect a crowd of other nervous, nametag-wearing applicants.

The Introduction

When you first get to the admissions office, you'll likely see a slide show introducing the school. Because this is the first thing, don't panic if you are unavoidably late. All you'll miss is an introduction, so don't let it throw you for the whole day. On the other hand, don't act overly casual about it either, as though you make a habit of being late. Assuming you show the proper amount of concern, no one takes a huge red marker and writes "late" on your application, so if you're poised, your interviewers will never know. That said, there is almost no reasonable excuse for being late, so plan to give yourself plenty of time.

Food, Glorious Food

Most med school interviews break for lunch after the tour and before the first interview. It's usually a free meal at the school cafeteria, often in the company of "host" med students. Try to relax and enjoy your meal, and don't forget to check your smile afterwards for leftovers.

The Tour

Med students who are conducting the tour may be evaluating you as well. Again, remember to treat every interaction as if it were a part of the interview. The medical student is getting a free day off work, so he or she will likely be very happy to chat with you. Find out from him or her, both directly and indirectly, if the medical school is for you. Ask questions like "How does the testing schedule affect your stress level?" "Do people in your class socialize together?" "What's the major hospital like?" "Do you feel safe walking to the parking deck at midnight?" and "What's the best/worst thing about this school?" Don't be aggressive or belligerent. If you've heard the school is not particularly welcoming to minorities, ask the question gently. Keep in mind that med students do tours because they like their school, and have some of the same loyal motivations as the volunteering faculty.

You can get a feel for the school by watching the medical students in the hospital portion of the tour. Do they look comfortable? Do they seem well oriented to the wards? How do they walk through the emergency department—do they waltz through or timidly invite you to look through the windows? These sorts of observations can give you hints about the type of clinical training the hospital gives, that is, hands on or by instruction.

Advice from the Inside

We asked an admissions committee member for some pointers on interview day. Here's what she told us:

- Be incredibly nice to the school admissions secretary. He can be your best ally or your worst nightmare.
- It's fine to bring in bags if your flight leaves immediately after the interview.
- Most schools offer coffee when you first arrive. Be aware that caffeine can make you nervous.

- Don't try to outdo the competition by comparing stats or namedropping while waiting in the "greeting" room.
- Don't be vocal about not wanting to go to that school, even casually. "This is my safety" can safely assure you won't get an offer.
- Do your homework and be prepared to ask questions.
- Ask the interview coordinator whether the interviews are "open" or "closed" and how long each interview should last (more about these issues later).

Preparing for the Interview

Many students go into their first few interviews completely unprepared, hoping to get the hang of it as they go along. This strategy is extremely unwise. You want to be able to anticipate the questions and formulate the key points of your responses. Doing this can help you maximize your potential for success.

Understanding the Dynamics

The interview experience is multidimensional. Obviously it is a time for the admissions committee to check you out, which means it's also a time for you to "show your stuff." However, you should also approach the interview day as a chance to determine whether or not you would want to attend that particular medical school, assuming you have multiple acceptances.

Given that your primary concern is getting in, it is important to think about the interview from the perspective of the person at the other side of the desk—the interviewer. At most schools, you will have two interviewers: One will usually be given by someone who sits on the committee, while the other will be a physician from the community, the residency program, or the faculty. Alternatively, many medical schools utilize med student interviewers, and a few use administrative personnel. Regardless of their affiliation with the medical school, both of your interviewers are volunteering their time, giving up at least an hour of clinical, research, administrative, or study time.

The interviewer's fundamental job is to determine whether or not you have the necessary interpersonal skills and characteristics required of a future physician. These interpersonal skills include, but are not limited to, communication skills, social awareness, empathy, and cultural competency. In the process of the interview, the interviewer will be asking herself, "Do I like this applicant?" and "Can I see myself teaching him as a medical student, consulting with her as a colleague, or referring family members to him as a patient?" If the answer is "no," and that opinion is echoed by the second interviewer, it is unlikely that you will be accepted.

Why would interviewers volunteer their time to interview prospective med students? There are a few reasons, most of them altruistic, including:

- Quality control over those entering the health care profession
- Interest in helping choose the best candidates to better the school's reputation
- Loyalty to the admissions committee's goals of getting the best possible class
- Curiosity about the upcoming batch of future doctors
- Desire to help certain candidate types for personal reasons (minorities, football players, etcetera)
- Interest in education
- Feeling of duty toward an alma mater or toward the profession

When It Doesn't Click

The overwhelming majority of those interviewing do so out of conviction. Those with really strong convictions join the admissions committee itself, rather than just volunteer to interview on occasion. There may, however, be the occasional community or faculty physician who likes the power dynamic or who wants to find someone like herself, the best tennis-playing biology major from Indiana. If your interviewer asks questions you don't think are appropriate or seems to be biased against you from the start, don't let it rattle you.

Many medical schools will end the interview day by asking you to complete a questionnaire concerning your interview experience. If you truly believe your interviewer was inappropriate, you may want to make note of it on your questionnaire. If you do, be specific as to your concerns, describing the incident in behavioral terms. Don't say, "Dr. X didn't seem interested in my application," when what you really mean is "After the first time Dr. X referred to me by wrong name, I corrected him. Unfortunately, this continued throughout the interview. As a result I was left wondering if he had me confused with another applicant." Alternatively, you may speak with an admissions office staff member regarding your concerns; she will advise you as to your options.

The Interviewer from Hell

Politics are rampant in all systems; chances are, if you get a weird feeling from the interview, the person interviewing is someone whom the committee can't politely refuse. For example, it may be well known at one school that Dr. X is abrasive and unwelcoming to students he interviews. If he is also a prestigious head of cardiology, it's possible that the committee couldn't refuse his interest, and takes his assessments with a grain of salt, hoping that the students interviewed by him aren't too turned off.

Learning Their Interests

At the beginning of the interview day you're likely to receive your personal schedule of events, including names of the doctors interviewing you and their titles or specialties. Some schools try to match you with interviewers who share your interests, but it may not always be possible. If you happen to know one of your interviewers by research or clinical reputation, great. But if you don't, forgo the temptation to run to the library to look up their publications or where they did their training. Chances are you won't have time; besides, it makes it look like you're trying to hard. Instead, we recommend you mull these things over while you await your interviews.

- Older doctors/heads of departments are more likely to be the ones on the admissions committee itself.
- Researchers are more likely to be interested and ask questions about your research, or about science.
- Generalists or younger doctors are more likely to ask personal questions (see below) or questions about how you'll approach the learning part of medical school, or personal "survival" characteristics (how you handle stress, whether you study or play well with others, etcetera).
- Administrators may be more likely to ask questions about ethics or your future plans as a doctor.

Typical Areas of Assessment

The faculty members at each medical school are charged with determining the institutional mission of their particular school and to that end, the qualities and characteristics upon which its medical students shall be selected. For this reason, it is impossible to know which characteristics the interview is designed to assess at each medical school to which you are granted an interview. However, the following are areas of appraisal in most interviews:

Intellectual Curiosity

It should come as no surprise that intellectual ability is an area of assessment throughout the application process. However, by the time you make it to the interview, it is generally recognized that you have the intellectual ability to negotiate the medical school curriculum. Therefore, what is being assessed at the interview is not so much your ability to do the work, but ways in which you approach the unknown. Do you do so openly, with curiosity? How do you organize your thoughts? What is your preferred style of learning? What learning experiences have you had outside of the traditional classroom setting? As a future physician, you will be required to learn continuously: from your patients, colleagues, scientific journals, as well as the world around you. It is imperative that you enjoy learning, that you have appropriate study habits, and that you have broad intellectual interests.

Social Awareness and Cultural Competency

As a future physician, your patients will come from backgrounds that are similar to and very different from your own. Therefore, the interview is used to assess the extent to which you have exposed yourself to people whose interests, religion, culture, economics, gender, age, ethnicity, language, education, and race are different from your own. What value do you place on these differences? It is important that for each of your patients you are able to modify your behavior in such a way as to show respect, inspire confidence, and motivate them to implement whatever changes they need to make to positively effect their health.

Communication and Interpersonal Skills

Again, the interviewer will be assessing your ability to interact with people who are different from you, whether they be your patients and their families, allied health personnel, or other physicians. Before you interview, it's important that you gain some awareness of yourself as a social being: What is your perception of the impression you make on others? What is your response when others have misunderstood your words or actions? What experiences have you had working or playing on a team? What is your response to criticism? As a future physician, it is imperative that you have the appropriate communication and interpersonal skills to interact successfully with others under dynamic and often emotionally charged conditions.

Maturity

Medicine is a very wonderful, but very difficult, career. It has often been said that it is not so much a profession as it is a calling. The interview is therefore used to explore your expectations of a medical career, as well as assess your maturity, your ability to cope with frustration, and your leadership skills. What efforts have you made to explore a health career? Have you experienced disappointment in your life? What are you most proud of? Under what circumstances do you become frustrated? What is your definition of a leader? In order to be a happy, successful physician it is important that your expectations be grounded in some reality, and that you have the necessary personality skills and characteristics required to cope with the challenges and stresses of being a physician.

Types of Interviews

There are four types of interview you're likely to encounter: open, semi-open, closed, and group.

Open

With these, the interviewer has already reviewed your application and personal statement. He or she will often begin the interview by referring to the application or a particular section of your personal statement.

Semi-Open

Here, the interviewer has read your personal statement, but nothing else. These interviews are likely to begin by relating to whatever event or opinion you put forth in your personal statement. If you didn't explicitly make much of it in your essay, the interview may begin with, "So how did you decide you wanted to be a doctor?"

Closed

Here, the interviewer has never seen your application folder. He or she may begin with a very open-ended question, such as "Tell me a little about yourself." The unfortunate side effect of the "closed" interview is that you feel you've put hours and hours into your application, only to have an interviewer ask questions easily answered by the first few sentences. Though you may be tempted to give a sarcastic response to "Tell me about yourself" out of frustration that your masterpiece went unread, avoid the urge. Answer pleasantly, and think before you go into an interview about how you'll launch into talking about yourself if the interviewer hasn't read your essay.

Group

These are the exception. In a group interview, you might have three interviewers and three interviewees in a room. After an introduction and a generic, "loosen up" question, each of the interviewers gets to ask questions to each interviewee. Given time constraints, there is usually just time for one question apiece from each of the interviewers, which may not be the same for each interviewee. (For example, Dr. Bob: "John, tell me more about your Space Shuttle experience. Mabel, how do you see your cold fusion experiments relating to medicine?") Group interviews are designed for a school to gauge how well you "play with others," and whether you can share airtime while being charming and eloquent, too.

> ### Tips for Groupies
>
> Etiquette tips for group interviews:
>
> - Don't hog the airtime
> - Refer to others' answers if you get the same question after them
> - Try not to take yourself too seriously

These days, most schools conduct "semi-open" or "closed" interviews to avoid something called the "halo effect." If an interviewer looks at your wonderful scores and grades, he or she runs the risk of thinking everything you say is wonderful, even if in person you're not that scintillating. The down side about the semi-open or closed interview is that the interviewer may not know everything he or she needs to know about your application in order to represent you adequately before the admissions committee. For example, if you bombed junior year, your interviewer may write you off without really listening to how you fed your family, went to school, and managed to save enough to do relief work in Uganda over the summer. Remember that one of your interviewer's primary responsibilities is to act as your advocate. If you are granted a semi-open or closed interview, it is up to you to bring to your interviewer's attention anything concerning your application that you believe requires further discussion. That way, the interviewer will be best able to address questions posed by the admissions committee about your application.

As was mentioned earlier, a typical interview will last anywhere from 30 to 45 minutes. However, it is not unheard of for a school to schedule interviews of 15 minutes or 90 minutes in length. This is an important piece of information for you to have before you begin the interview, so ask the interview coordinator how long interviews generally last at that particular medical school. How you prioritize the topics you would like to cover during the interview will be very different if you are anticipating the interview to last 15, 45, or 90 minutes.

How to Prepare

As we said before, don't even think about going into your interviews cold. You need to prepare well in advance. You'll need to think about not only what you may encounter once you're facing your inter- viewer, but also when you'll interview, how you'll get there, how you'll behave, and what you'll wear.

Your best resources when preparing for the interview will include your premed advisor, students cur- rently attending the medical school, and the school of medicine's catalog.

Scheduling

Your interview invitations will probably arrive at approximately the same time. Remember, the sooner you have your interview, the sooner you'll be considered for acceptance. Schedule the interviews as early as possible. Many students will try to schedule interviews at less competitive schools earlier, to gain interview experience and overcome early jitters. However, don't postpone your other interviews too long, as it will delay completion of your applications.

Financial reasons may compel you to try to schedule groups of interviews in particular geographical regions. For instance, you may want to set up a West Coast interview tour and visit several schools in the same area during one trip.

If you get one interview in a far-flung region and haven't yet heard from another school in the same place, don't hesitate to give the second school a call. Politely ask, "I'll be in this region on such and such a date interviewing at So and So. If you are planning to interview me, would it be possible to schedule an appointment near that time so I can make only one plane trip?" Schools will usually ask to get back to you, go look at your file, and then tell you yes if they are planning to interview you. If they're already booked for that time, they may offer another time slot.

Travel and Accommodations

It is at this point that the whole application process can really begin to get expensive. You probably know that you can keep costs down by making airline reservations as far in advance as possible and staying over a Saturday. But did you know that major airlines often offer discounts to applicants for interview travel? Check with your premed advisor or premed club for details. It might also be worth your while to check with discount travel agents. They frequently have discounted tickets for sale, even if you only have a few days notice. One other air travel tip: Carry your luggage with you on the plane. The last thing you want on interview day is to have your luggage sent to the wrong place.

Always do research in advance to find out about parking or the best way to reach the med school from the airport. Usually, your interview offer will include directions to the school and information on accommodations. Many medical schools have programs allowing you to stay with a med student for

Word of Mouth

Check out a nifty little Web site maintained by Johns Hopkins: http://interviewfeedback.com/meded/, in which recently interviewed applicants complete an online questionnaire regarding their interview experience at particular medical schools.

free. Although a complementary room may be economically enticing, remember that it's important for you to be comfortable. If sleeping on the floor of a medical student's apartment is going to stress you out, you'd be better off staying at the nearest budget motel.

On the other hand, if money is short and you can find a student with an extra bed, it may be a good opportunity to get an inside scoop on the school's personality. Also, just as the medical student touring you around can give you great information and can affect how you view the school, someone you stay with can have an impact on your admission. Since he or she is doing the admissions office a favor by agreeing to be willing host, the office secretary will listen to that person's feedback, such as, "Hey, that last guy was really great! He'd be good to have in the class." It therefore behooves you to treat your host with respect. Remember you are a guest in his home. Don't be demanding, don't expect him to act as a taxi service, don't hog all the hot water for your shower in the morning, and remember to clean up after yourself.

If at all possible, try to arrive the night before the interview in order to familiarize yourself with the area and the school. This allows you to avoid travel delays the day of your interview, and will also give you the opportunity to unwind and get a good night's sleep.

Dress

The interview is not the time to make a fashion statement. Whether you like it or not, your physical appearance will be the first impression you make on the interviewer. You want to be remembered as the self-confident candidate with loads of charm and wit, not the one with the funny hat or braided facial hair.

Men should opt for a dark suit (blue, gray, black) and an attractive, but not too flashy, tie. Your tie should be a real one, not a clip on (you don't want it falling off in your lap during the interview), and unless you're already experienced in this area, this is probably not the time to start experimenting with a bow tie. Facial hair should be groomed, and you should probably forgo the earring even if you normally wear one (but it's up to you). Sneakers are definitely out.

Women should wear a suit or dressy coordinates. If you opt for a dress or skirt, watch your hem length. Remember a short hemline may become inappropriately short when you sit and cross your legs. Your shoes should be closed-toed. Go easy on the jewelry and makeup, and you should probably forego the perfume altogether. Stay away from dangling earrings and plunging necklines. If you haven't packed an extra pair of nylons in your purse, it's better to wear a pair that matches your skin tone in case you get a run. Also, dress to tour: Uncomfortable shoes won't help you show yourself at your best. You may want to bring a leather folder or binder for the extra packets of information they give you, but don't bring a briefcase unless you have to.

Be prepared for whatever the weather brings. If it is expected to be hot and humid, wear a blouse or shirt that you wouldn't mind being seen if you were to take your jacket off. If there is a possibility of rain in the forecast, carry an umbrella and wear a coat. Snow? Opt for a sweater instead of a blouse or shirt, add some gloves, and don't forget your coat.

Finally, one suit or dress is usually enough. You don't have to change outfits for every interview. In fact, when you go to your interviews, you'll begin to recognize certain of your fellow candidates by their interview outfits. It doesn't matter. Remember that you're trying to impress your interviewer, not your competition. If you have a bunch of interviews in a row, make arrangements for dry cleaning your beloved interview outfit.

Sharpening Your Skills

You can get yourself psyched up for the interview by giving yourself a "trial run," anticipating the questions you'll be asked, and understanding what you might encounter on interview day.

Mock Interviews

Mock interviews are invaluable trial runs. You finally have a chance to answer some of those practice questions. You can have someone evaluate your speaking style, the content of your answers, your body language, and your overall presentation.

> ### *Candid Camera*
>
> If you're able to videotape yourself in a mock interview, try playing the tape back in fast forward. Any nervous gestures you display will seem even more obvious (and comical) when they repeat every two seconds.

Some colleges offer mock interviews. Check the availability of these by consulting your premed advisor or career center. In any case, even if a formal mock interview is not available, you can always have a friend or relative act as the interviewer and evaluate your performance. You may even want to videotape your interview for a more detailed critique. Regardless of which route you take, be sure to wear your interview outfit. As corny as this sounds, you need to practice wearing your professional attire, which unfortunately isn't like wearing your favorite pair of jeans. Not only do you need to get used to the feel of your new clothes, but if you're going to suddenly develop a nervous tick, chances are it will somehow be related to your interview clothes. If this happens, it's better to discover and correct it during your practice interview, not during the real thing.

After your mock interview, be sure to solicit feedback. Only then will you realize if you speak too quickly, should enunciate more clearly, have a tendency to play with your tie or skirt hem when you are nervous, or start every sentence with "like," "umm," or "you know."

Common Interview Questions

More often than not, the interviewer will base his or her questions on your personal statement and application. But on occasion, you might be asked to comment on a medically related current event or ethical issue. Since you're planning to become a doctor, these questions are fair game. It's not expected, however, that you'll be an expert on these topics, just that you'll have thought about them and have something reasonably intelligent to share. Read the newspaper and keep up on current events. Go through some back issues of a news weekly and read all the pertinent medically related articles.

Here are some classic interview questions:

Personal

- Tell me about yourself.
- What do you do for fun?
- Why have you decided to pursue medicine as a career?
- When did you decide that you wanted to be a doctor?
- Do you have any family members who are physicians?
- What is your greatest strength/weakness? success/failure?
- If you don't get into medical school, what will you do?
- What did you like about college?
- What is your favorite book? What are you reading now?
- What area of medicine are you interested in?
- Where do you see yourself in ten years? (Hint: Don't say "prison.")
- Where else have you applied? Why do you want to go here?
- What leadership roles have you assumed?
- What clinical experience have you had?

Ethical

- What are your views on abortion?
- Do you have an opinion on fetal-tissue research?
- How would you feel about treating a patient infected with HIV?
- Do you agree with Dr. Kevorkian's actions?
- How do you feel about treating uninsured or indigent patients?

Hypothetical Situations

- You are treating a terminally ill patient who is being kept alive by life support. You feel that he should be taken off the machines. What do you do?
- A pregnant teenager comes to you to discuss her options. She hasn't told her parents about her pregnancy. What do you do?

Health-Care Issues

- What's the biggest problem facing medicine today?
- What do you think the role of the government should be in health care?
- Do you think health care is a right or a privilege?
- Have you been following the health-care debate? Where do you stand?
- How do you feel about socialized medicine? the Canadian and British Health systems?
- Do you know what an HMO is? a PPO?

Obviously, you won't encounter all of the above questions. Additionally, there may be others that you're asked that aren't on this list. If you take the time to examine these issues, you'll have the confidence to answer most questions that come your way. Practice answering these questions, but do not memorize answers or practice monologues in front of the mirror. An interview is a conversation; you're not auditioning for *Hamlet*. Nothing is worse than answers that sound canned. You must be able to improvise and think on your feet.

Anticipating the "Why"

Admissions committees don't want to know the "what" of your answers as much as the "why." For example, if you're asked what you're most proud of, and the answer is running a marathon, you might want to extrapolate by saying something like, "I had never been athletic, but as I researched health and medical school, I realized that exercise really matters. I decided that my future patients would benefit from me practicing the exercise I'll preach, so I started running. I was also feeling like I needed to prove to myself that I had the discipline for medical school, so I decided to commit to running a marathon."

Address Your Weaknesses

"If an applicant has anything on his or her résumé that might raise eyebrows, I would encourage him or her to write to the admissions committee addressing the apparent weakness. I flunked my chemistry course in my freshman year of college. I retook chemistry after college and got excellent grades, but there was no hiding the F on my undergraduate transcript. I sent out letters addressing this to every school I applied to and was commended for my honesty and maturity in doing so."

—Laura Hodes, Columbia University College of Physicians and Surgeons; adapted from Newsweek/Kaplan's *How to Choose a Career and Graduate School*

When you're asked a personal question, make sure your answer is—and sounds—honest. Nothing sounds worse than a corny, altruistic revision of an event. If the "why" of an answer is unrelated to medicine, that's fine.

Managing the Interview Day

You'll probably be more than a little nervous on interview day. Here are some tips to help you make the experience more manageable.

Before the Interview

- Arrive early if you can. Nothing is worse than being late to an interview, so make sure to give yourself plenty of time to get there. Don't be rushed.
- Don't bring family members or girlfriends/boyfriends to the interview. Drop them at the mall; give them movie money. Just don't take them to your interview!
- Be sure to review your application and your personal statement before you arrive. The interviewer may ask you specific questions concerning your application and personal statement. Bring a copy with you as well.
- After arriving at the admissions office, be sure to be polite to the receptionist or other support staff. A rude comment or inappropriate behavior can quickly be passed on to admissions committee members and interviewers.
- Treat every interaction as if it were an integral part of the interview.

During the Interview

- Acknowledge the interviewer by name ("Hello, Dr. X"), and introduce yourself.
- Shake hands (firm, but not bone crunching).
- Maintain eye contact.
- Don't fidget.
- Don't cross arms.
- Don't touch any items on the interviewer's desk.
- Try not to speak too quickly.
- Smile at appropriate times.
- Avoid being arrogant and dogmatic. Remember you're not a doctor yet. You don't know what medical school or medicine is really like. At the same time, do not compromise your views in order to please the interviewer. Be firm, but flexible.
- If the interviewer is being antagonistic, do not answer in kind. Think before you speak. Do not raise your voice. Speak slowly. Be cool and composed.
- If you don't know the answer to a specific question, don't be afraid to say that you don't know. If you try to make something up, the interviewer will see right through you. This could

simply be a composure test. It takes a great deal of maturity to simply say, "I don't know." (Of course, you can't answer "I don't know" if the question is "Tell me about yourself.")

After the Interview

- Shake hands and say good-bye.
- In some instances, you may want to write your interviewer a thank-you note. In that case, be sure to obtain the address of the interviewer through the admissions office. A card or short note is appropriate (but no novelty greeting cards, please). Try to mention something specific about your interview.
- You can express your continued interest in the school, but don't grovel. The truth is that the thank-you note probably won't make any difference in your candidacy.

CHAPTER 11

The Admissions Process: An Inside View

As noted earlier, for every three applicants to medical school, only one gets in. For the more competitive schools, the odds are much slimmer. Since so many med students are seemingly qualified—good GPA's, respectable MCAT scores, prerequisites in place—how do med schools make the cut? What are the factors that really count?

Initial Review

The first criteria for getting an interview and an offer is, "Can the student do the work?" You'll prove you're capable of medical school level work primarily with your grades and MCAT scores. Some admissions officers will candidly say they have a formula, such as GPA × "school difficulty conversion factor" × MCAT score. Many have soft cutoffs that differ for in- and out-of-state candidates, and that are mediated by extenuating circumstances described in the personal statement or premed cover letter. Remember, one of the reasons many schools get lots of secondaries is to get the fullest possible point of view on an applicant before making a decision.

The first cut will eliminate those who fall below the school's typical standards for both GPA and MCAT. Left are those who have sufficient proof of their academic ability. The weighting of the two depends on a number of different things.

GPA

How your GPA is viewed is colored by where you went to school, the particular classes you took, if your grades are inflated, and if there are any other mitigating circumstances.

Difficulty of the Classes

Princeton University, for example, is known in admissions circles to have a grueling organic chemistry class, for which a C may represent perfectly good work. Especially if you are applying to schools near your undergraduate alma mater, you can expect that the local admissions officers are acquainted with the professors and difficulty of the classes. They can look at individual class grades and interpret how much harder you had to work for the B in P-Chem than for that A in Advanced Anthropological Debates. That said, passing the first-round draft requires you do have a certain level of GPA. More of the specific evaluation of your classes occurs after you've gotten past the interviews.

School Selectivity

One way in which schools can determine the value of your GPA is with the *Comparative Guide to American Colleges,* which ranks schools from "Most Selective" on down. This enables medical committees to view your GPA with regard to how tough your school really was.

Grade Inflation

The committees also consider grade inflation, which is prevalent at many schools. Committee members usually know which institutions tend to inflate and which don't, and they take that into account when evaluating your particular GPA.

Foreign Study

A few students every year run into problems because the majority of their undergraduate equivalent education was not done in this country. English and Irish educational systems, for example, do not curve grades. This means that a student ranked third in a class of 500 at a highly selective institution can have a GPA of 2.3. If you've done your undergrad work outside of the States, have a school official include class rank with the transcript. You can also ask for a letter from the dean, detailing what percentage of students get, for example, a mark equivalent to 70 percent, to show that your 74 percent put you at the top of the class. Finally, make sure your letters of recommendation (in English) mention your performance compared to that of your classmates, and the selectivity of the program.

Narrative Evaluations

If your school uses narrative course evaluations rather than grades, admissions committee members will convert these evaluations into grades if you're to be considered further. Since this is not always a straightforward process, consider requesting a letter grade instead of an evaluation, particularly for prerequisite courses.

Trend

Some medical schools consider a positive trend in your GPA over time. If you got off to a slow start but have improved significantly in later semesters, take heart. On the other hand, if your grades have been dropping you may have a problem. These schools believe that a GPA of 3.5 arrived at by GPA's of 3.0, 3.5, and 4.0 in your freshman, sophomore, and junior years respectively differ markedly from a 3.5 earned by a 4.0, 3.5, 3.0 sequence.

MCAT Scores

Because the GPA is subject to such variability and interpretation, the MCAT score has taken on more predominance in past years. The three MCAT scores—Verbal Reasoning, Physical Sciences, and Biological Sciences, each of which yields a score between 1 and 15—are used to give the admissions committee a nationally standardized view of your science background, reasoning ability, and future potential. A fourth "letter" score assesses writing ability.

How They're Used

MCAT scores can be viewed in different ways. Some schools add the three scores and consider this as one combined value, while others consider each score separately.

Verbal Reasoning, designed to test your logical ability, thinking skills, and ability to evaluate information, is often viewed as a gauge of your overall intelligence and ability to communicate. And while science scores are usually seen as measures of your abilities in particular sciences, they are also compared to your grades in those subjects.

How the writing sample section is intended, and how it is actually used by most med schools, are two different things. AAMC designed it to gauge your written communication ability, as well as your proficiency at following directions. They intended for schools to read the essay if they wanted additional information about the student's writing ability. In practice, this portion of the MCAT often receives far less notice than the other three.

Neglected Writing Sample

Inundated with more applications than ever before, most schools simply don't have the staff to make extensive use of the writing sample. It's more common for admissions committees to use the personal statement to gauge your writing ability.

Taking It More Than Once

The AMCAS summary page lists your most recent MCAT score, the second-most recent score, and a reading for the total number of MCATs taken. Taking the test more than once can work in your favor if you improve, but it can be a black mark if you do poorly in a particular subject more than once. If your first test results indicate a weak area, make sure you prepare well before you take the test a second time.

Officially, you can take the MCAT only three times. However, to take it a fourth, you need only send a rejection letter from a medical school so you can demonstrate that you are still trying to get in. Think twice about doing this, though—taking the test that many times casts into question your ability to do medical school work.

The Secondary Review

As the admissions committee reviews your secondary application, its focus begins to shift from your intellectual abilities to your nonacademic accomplishments. It is at the secondary stage that you may be asked to submit letters of recommendation, a list of your extracurricular activities, a second essay on a designated topic, and any number of additional materials.

Who Gets a Secondary?

Some medical schools send secondary applications to only a fraction of the applicant pool, while other medical schools send secondary applications to virtually all applicants. What does it mean if you have received a secondary? If the school "prescreens," then you know that you have been found to be academically competitive and are somewhat comparable academically to the other applicants also receiving a secondary. If the school does not prescreen prior to sending out secondaries, the fact that you have received one doesn't tell you much. If you want to determine your statistical chances of receiving an interview after receipt of a secondary application, it is possible to do so by comparing the number of applicants receiving secondary applications to the number of applicants receiving an interview at any given school; you can find this information in the School Profiles section of the MSAR.

Understanding the Process

You can learn a great deal about how the admissions process works at an individual medical school by reviewing that school's secondary application, which should be available at your school's premed office. Unlike the AMCAS application, which is a generic application used by most medical schools, the secondary application is the individual medical school's own work, created by that school. Therefore, you are only asked to address issues that are relevant to that particular school's admissions process. For instance, if on its secondary application a particular medical school asks you for a great deal of information concerning your extracurricular activities, it's a pretty safe bet that extracurriculars are counted in its screening process.

Conversely, if you aren't asked about your extracurricular activities, they are probably not considered important to that institution. If you are asked whether a relative, no matter how distant, attended their college or university, you can be pretty certain you'll get "brownie points" if you can answer in the affirmative; it's likely that they're looking for family "legacies." Other schools make no mention of family connections because they're not relevant to the process.

Criminal Convictions

You may be asked on a secondary application if you have a criminal record. While the AMCAS application does not ask about history of criminal convictions, more and more medical schools are beginning to do so on the secondary application. Some medical schools limit the type of convictions that applicants must report to felonies, while other medical schools broaden the scope to include traffic violations and misdemeanors.

Because criminal behavior says something about a candidate's veracity and integrity (both of which are critically important characteristics in a physician), medical school admissions committees view prior criminal convictions very seriously.

Unless the particular state in which a medical school is located prohibits a physician with a conviction of a specific offense from obtaining a license, then conviction of that specific offense, in and of itself, will not prohibit an applicant from gaining acceptance to medical schools in the state. Admissions committees look at each situation on a case-by-case basis and view the behavior holistically, considering mitigating factors leading up to and surrounding the conviction as well as the individual's perspective on the incident. For this reason, two admissions committees may view the same incident or applicant differently, and the same behavior committed by two different applicants may be viewed differently by the same committee.

Tell Them Yourself

As with all aspects of your medical school application, you should be forthright when discussing prior convictions. Information of all sorts has a mysterious way of falling into the lap of admissions committees. If a committee learns of previous criminal or unethical behavior from a source other than the applicant, chances of that applicant's admission are virtually nil.

Secondary Fee

In most cases, you must pay a fee when you submit a secondary application. While a small number of schools do not have a fee, the majority charge between 40 and 60 dollars, but some go as high as $125. The School Profiles section of the MSAR contains information regarding the amount of each medical school's secondary fee. If you are unable to afford the fee, contact the admissions office concerning its fee waiver policy. Many medical schools will waive their secondary fee if you received a fee waiver through AMCAS, while other medical schools have their own fee waiver policy.

The Interview and Beyond

Your application is complete, and you've had a wonderful interview. What happens now?

At this point, both the expertise of the admissions committee and sheer luck come into play. One important element that is beyond your control is whether you are the candidate who fits the profile that a particular medical school needs at that particular moment. If you are, the admissions committee may quickly decide to accept you. If you're not, however, you are on equal footing with many other applicants who are as qualified as you are, and who have also had strong interviews. If you have someone on the admissions committee who is particularly taken with you, your chances increase. If you don't have a champion on the committee, or if there is nothing remarkably distinctive in your application, however strong it is, you may be waitlisted—or rejected.

Importance of the Interview

An invitation to interview at any medical school means you're acceptable on paper. That's the good news. The bad news is, so is everyone else being interviewed. The interview adds the only new piece of information, and therefore has the potential to become the deciding factor.

After your interview, your interviewers will submit a written statement to the admissions committee concerning their assessment of your candidacy for medical school in general and for their medical school in particular.

At all medical schools, if you have a poor interview, you will almost certainly be rejected. That is how important the interview is. It is also an indication of how important admissions committees believe personal characteristics are in the making of a great physician.

> ## *"False Positive"*
>
> Interviews can result in a "false positive" impression. The fact that an applicant can behave in a socially appropriate manner for a 30-minute interview really means nothing more than that he or she can behave in a socially appropriate manner for 30 minutes at a time. It does not mean that the person he or she seemed to be in the interview is the person he or she really is.

At most medical schools, a particularly strong interview may ensure your acceptance. However, there are a few medical schools at which the results of the interview come into play only if they are negative. At those schools, as at all others, a negative interview results in the applicant's rejection. But the results of a positive interview there are not considered, and the applicant falls back to his or her pre-interview ranking. These schools reason that all applicants know they should be on their best behavior, and most will be able to behave in a socially appropriate manner for a 30-minute interview. If an applicant cannot pull this off, either he is completely out of touch with social norms, or simply doesn't care. In either case, these are not personality traits that are desirable in a future physician.

Nonetheless, most admissions committees count the interview for positive as well as negative impressions. After reviewing the entire application, including the interviewers' comments and recommendations, the committee votes on the candidacy of each applicant. The vote may be a yes/no vote; it may be an immediate accept/wait list/reject vote; or it may be a numerical score indicating each committee member's individual level of support for that applicant. As a result of the committee vote, candidates will either receive an immediate acceptance, rejection, or will be placed on the alternate list, otherwise known as the wait list.

What Is the Admissions Committee?

The Liaison Committee on Medical Education (LCME), the body that accredits medical schools, states that the selection of medical students is the responsibility of the medical school faculty through a duly constituted committee. That committee is commonly referred to as the Admissions Committee. The LCME permits others to assist with the evaluation of applicants, but does not permit the final responsibility to be delegated outside of the faculty. In other words, medical schools are required to have a faculty admissions committee that may have nonfaculty members. The schools are given wide latitude in the size and composition of that committee.

Size and Composition

Admissions committees vary in size from the very small (8–10 members) to the very large (75 or more members). At some schools, especially those with very large committees, there may be a number of sub-committees, each charged with reviewing a segment of the applicant pool. Applications may be distributed alphabetically, by region, or by the undergraduate college the applicants attended. There may be a separate committee or subcommittee to review MSTP or M.D./Ph.D. applicants or applicants for other special programs. Another approach is to have an Executive Committee that guides the work of the sub-committees.

At most medical schools, the majority of Admissions Committee members are members of the faculty from either clinical or basic science departments. Schools try to balance committee membership by age, gender, departmental affiliation, and ethnic background. Many schools also have one or more medical student members. The student members may have full voting rights or may be advisory to the committee. Some schools include one or more representatives of the affiliated undergraduate college. Representatives of the general public also serve on some schools' admissions committees.

Duties of an Admissions Committee Member

All admissions committee members share one basic responsibility, the selection of applicants for admission. At many schools the committee members' duties go well beyond just making final decisions. For example, they may also participate in the initial review of applications to determine which applicants will be asked to submit supplemental materials or which students to invite for interviews. Frequently, admissions committee members conduct admissions interviews, and at some schools they are the only ones who interview. On the other hand, some schools do not permit admissions committee members to interview any applicants.

How Admissions Committees Work

With 125 medical schools in the United States, it is likely that there are nearly that many different ways in which admissions committees arrive at their final decisions. There are, however, some relatively common approaches, which we will discuss below.

In one approach, applications may be discussed during a meeting of the committee. In this model, either a committee member or an admissions office staff member "presents" the application. Details of the application are described by the presenter with discussion following the presentation. The person who interviewed the applicant may be the presenter or may be present and join in the discussion. A vote may be taken following the discussion, or committee members may assign a score to the application, with the applicants receiving the highest scores being admitted. Advocates of this method believe that the open discussion of applications is essential to arriving at the best decisions. Opponents argue that a particularly vocal committee member can skew the votes of others and have an undue influence on the decision process.

Other schools use a rule-based approach in which committee members review and award points to each part of the application (GPA, MCAT scores, interview, personal comments, recommendations, out of class activities, etcetera) based on a predetermined scoring system, or rule. The applicants with the highest scores are admitted. Advocates of this system point to the inherent fairness of treating each part of the application the same for all applicants and reducing the advocacy effect of particularly vocal committee members. Opponents say that it minimizes the judgment each committee member can bring to the process and eliminates valuable discussion between committee members.

Schools using a holistic approach have several members of the committee read and score the application as a whole. Each reader brings his or her own knowledge, experience, and judgment to the process. Schools using this method believe that because the reader has access to the entire application and the freedom to score the application as a whole, he or she can judge the file as a whole. The use of multiple

How Do They Decide?

Admissions Committees most commonly use the following approaches to arrive at their final decisions:

- Open discussion of all candidates, followed by vote

- Rule-based system in which each section of the application is scored separately

- Holistic system in which the entire application is read and scored as a whole

readers adds collective judgment to the evaluation of applications. Supporters of this approach cite the value of collective judgment, the opportunity for committee members to weigh the parts of applications differently depending on circumstances, and to thoroughly review all application parts. Opponents point out the danger of inconsistently weighing criteria and the absence of discussion as weaknesses of this method.

Alternate Lists

Applicants have a love-hate relationship with the alternate lists. Learning that they have been placed on the alternate list brings most applicants feelings of relief ("Thank goodness I wasn't rejected"), followed by feelings of disappointment ("What do you mean you aren't accepting me at this time!"), which ultimately culminate in feelings of frustration ("Won't someone tell me what my chances are?"). These feelings are compounded by the fact that medical schools use their alternate lists differently, and for the most part are reticent about divulging specific information regarding an applicant's status.

How the Alternate List Works

There are two basic ways alternate lists may be utilized. In the first, the list is very fluid. Interviewed applicants are constantly added to the list after they clear the admissions committee, while accepted applicants are skimmed off the top. In the second method, the alternate list is used as a large holding category for the applicants who are not accepted with the initial round of acceptees. These two basic methods are further complicated by the fact that some medical schools rank applicants on the alternate list, while others do not.

How an individual medical school uses its alternate list is largely influenced by its acceptance policies. All medical schools ultimately need to accept more students than are reflected in the actual class size. This is because many successful applicants receive multiple acceptances and therefore have to turn down all but one school, leaving the "rejected" schools to offer new acceptances. Admissions committees have an historical perspective as to how many acceptances they must offer to fill the medical school class. Depending on the school's admissions policies, the dean of admissions may send out enough acceptances to initially fill the class, and wait for withdrawals to occur before sending out additional acceptances. As an example, imagine that medical school "X" has a class size of 100. In the past, this school has made between 230–250 offers of acceptance to fill each class. In this admission scenario, the first 100 acceptances would be sent out. Further acceptances are not sent until a position is declined by one of the original accepted applicants. Then, and only then, would an additional offer of acceptance be sent. This process would continue until the class matriculated in the fall. Under this process, movement on the alternate list is fluid, with applicants constantly drawn from the pool to fill openings as they occur. As a result, alternates may begin receiving acceptances as early as the spring.

Alternatively, the dean of admissions may decide to accept most if not all of those applicants that the admissions committee finds to be immediately acceptable, even if it results in the potential overfilling of the class. Imagine that the admissions committee of medical school "X" found 200 applicants to be immediately acceptable. The dean of admissions sends all of them acceptances knowing that it generally takes 230–250 offers of acceptance to fill its 100-person class. She therefore feels comfortable sending out 200 acceptances right off the bat, knowing that she is still under the total number of acceptances ultimately sent in any given year to fill the class. Now, the dean waits for an opening to occur before new offers of acceptance are made to people on the alternate list. But at this point, 101 accepted applicants must withdraw before the first opening is created and the first alternate accepted. Under this scenario, alternates do not typically hear about an acceptance until shortly before the class matriculates.

Unfortunately, most medical schools are somewhat reluctant to discuss an applicant's chances of being accepted from the alternate list. This may be because the alternate list is unranked, or because no one really knows how many applicants will be accepted from the alternate list in any given year.

Important Dates in the Waiting Game

With the exception of Early Decision Programs, AMCAS medical schools do not offer acceptances prior to October 15 of the application year. Note that this is the earliest date for acceptances; many medical schools do not offer acceptances prior to December or even January.

By March 15, AMCAS medical schools are supposed to have offered a number of acceptances equal to the size of their entering class. This would mean that med school "X" must have offered 100 acceptances (its class size) by March 15.

> ## *Mark Down These Dates*
>
> The following dates apply to AMCAS schools only:
>
> - October 15: earliest date for acceptances
>
> - March 15: date by which schools must have accepted enough students to fill their entering classes
>
> - May 15: applicants with multiple acceptances must decide on a school; more slots then become available

AMCAS recommends that applicants be allowed to hold multiple acceptances prior to May 15. But AMCAS schools adhering to these guidelines are, in the words of the MSAR, "free to apply appropriate rules for dealing with accepted applicants who, without adequate explanation, hold one or more places in other schools." This means that without specific permission of the individual medical schools to which an applicant is holding multiple acceptances, the affected medical school(s) may individually choose to rescind their offer of acceptance.

If you find yourself unable to make a decision between your schools prior to May 15, contact the individual medical schools at which you've been accepted and ask for a deadline extension. It is entirely within their prerogative to approve, or disapprove, such an extension. Ignore the May 15 date at your own risk.

Because AMCAS medical schools are theoretically filled by March 15, and applicants are free to hold multiple acceptances until May 15, the interim two months is a very slow period for new acceptances. With the passage of May 15, a significant number of positions become available. The acceptance process continues throughout the summer as openings occur.

Applicants may continue to receive new acceptances after May 15. When this happens, they must decide between the acceptances they are currently holding and the new acceptance just received. New acceptances may be received up until the time the applicant matriculates in medical school.

Swaying Your Case

If you're placed on a school's waiting list, you still have a chance to sway your case. One tactic you might think of taking is submitting an additional letter of recommendation. If someone offered to write you a letter but you didn't take him or her up on it, now might be the time to accept that offer. The letter might give the admissions committee additional information that can swing the balance; besides, the fact that you've sent something extra indicates that you're really interested in that particular medical school. Of course, the letter should be glowing, and the more facets the author has seen of your professional side, the better. If the recommender offered to write the letter, make sure the person mentions that it was his or her idea. Integrity and honesty are important here: The letter should be truthful, and not terribly overstated.

CHAPTER 12

What If You Get Rejected?

In 1999, approximately 38,500 applicants competed for the nation's 16,200 first-year medical school positions. Put another way, about 42 percent of the applicants who applied for the entering class of 1998 received an acceptance. For those who didn't, rejection was undoubtedly painful. However, if you have been rejected from medical school, that shouldn't stop you from applying at least a second time. According to the Association of American Medical Colleges, in 1999, nearly 46 percent of all first-time applicants were accepted, whereas those who applied a second time had an acceptance rate of approximately 35 percent—an encouraging statistic.

What Went Wrong?

Despite the promising statistics concerning acceptance rates of reapplicants, you shouldn't be lulled into thinking that all you need to do is reapply. You don't get points for perseverance. One of three broad areas must change in order for you to be successful in your reapplication efforts:

• Your application credentials must improve

• The applicant pool must become less competitive

• The profile of the applicant being sought by a particular medical school much change to fit your application

Don't Give Up

"If you think this is what you want to do, you might meet a lot of obstacles, but don't give up. If you want it bad enough, you will find a way to make it work. And it will be worth it."

—University of Alabama med student

Improving Your Application Credentials

The only one of these things you have any control over is your application. Therefore, before investing the time, energy, and money it takes to reapply, you need to identify those areas of your application that need improving. This involves each of the following steps:

- Talk to your premedical adviser

- Check with the schools you applied to

- Conduct a thorough self-analysis

- Consider the alternatives

- Develop a plan of action

Talk to Your Premedical Adviser

Your adviser is the person most likely to have good sense of your credentials and how they compare to those of applicants from your college who have been successful in getting into med school in the past. He or she may also be able to suggest reapplication strategies that other students have used successfully.

Check with the Medical Schools That Rejected You

Many medical schools will give you the opportunity to talk to someone from the admissions office about your application. You should particularly try to talk to schools that interviewed you to find out if they will discuss aspects of your application that the admissions committee found to be weak. You don't need to talk to the dean; most members of the admissions staff will be able to discuss their school's needs for their class, and how your application fits into the big picture.

> ### *Rely on the Experts*
>
> Be wary of well-meaning but uninformed advice from friends or others who have no connection to the medical school admissions process. This includes medical students and others who may have an association with a medical school but who have not had direct involvement in the review of applications.

After getting feedback from the schools you applied to, summarize their comments. Be careful not to get caught up in the minutiae. Keep your perspective. There is no governing body that stands over all the medical schools and dictates admissions policies. Rather, the faculty at each institution determines the qualities and characteristics upon which the student body is selected. Therefore, it is entirely possible that what one admissions committee is looking for in a potential medical student is entirely the opposite of what another medical school is selecting for. You need to see the big picture. Your premed adviser will probably be able to help in this regard. Look for those aspects of your application that most medical schools believed needed strengthening. Disregard comments that were made by only one or two people.

Conduct a Thorough Self-Analysis

Examine each element of your application in the same way that an admissions committee member would. Start with your academic record. How does it compare to those of applicants admitted recently? In 1999, 80 percent of admitted applicants had GPAs of 3.26 or above. If your overall and/or science GPA is below this level, it is likely that your academic record needs improvement. Remember, though, that this is the national average and that the range of acceptable grades varies widely from school to school.

Grades

Look at the trend in your grades over time. Have your grades been steady, improving, or dropping? An improving trend over time may be a sign that some additional strong coursework will be helpful while a sharply dropping trend may be a sign of a more serious problem.

MCAT Scores

Take a hard look at your MCAT scores. Avoid summing the three multiple-choice sections. Rather, look at each section separately to identify areas that need improvement, if any. Averages for students admitted in 1999 were: Verbal Reasoning, 9.5; Physical Sciences, 10.0; and Biological Sciences, 10.2. The standard deviations range from 1.7 to 1.9. The median Writing Sample score for admitted students was P. As with grades, the range of acceptable MCAT scores varies widely from school to school. Read the section on retaking the MCAT that appears further in this chapter to help determine whether you should sit for the test again.

Extracurricular Activities

Do your extracurricular activities reflect your interest in health care? Remember that admissions officers identified knowledge of health care and health care experience as among the most important factors considered in admissions. Do your activities show that you are the kind of multifaceted person that medical schools seek? As one admissions officer put it, "I look at what the applicant did when nobody was making him or her do anything, when nobody was looking." Medical schools are looking for more than good students. They want a wide variety of interesting people in their classes.

On the other hand, does your record of out-of-class activities indicate that you were overextended? To claim that your relatively low grades should be excused because you had too many activities will generally fall on deaf ears. Admissions committee members will likely conclude that you exercised poor judgment in setting your priorities.

Personal Statement

We discussed the personal statement in chapter 9. Read that chapter again and then look at your personal statement with a critical eye. Are you comfortable that an admissions committee member reading your statement would get to know something about you as a person and why you want to be a physician? What kind of picture of yourself did you paint?

Letters of Recommendation

Letters of recommendations can be hard to assess because you have not seen them. If you followed the advice given in chapter 7 and discussed your request for a letter with those writing your letters, the chances are that those letters were supportive. If your premedical committee submitted a letter on your behalf, you may be able to get some sense of its level of support when you meet with your premedical adviser. Be open to constructive feedback. This is not the time for confrontation.

Interview

Were you invited for any interviews? If not, this may be an indication that your application did not pass the academic/MCAT screen. Another possibility is that you applied to the wrong schools. If you did get some interviews, how did they go? Were you prepared? Were you able to answer the interviewers questions and participate in an engaging dialogue? How did you feel after the interview was completed? Although it is hard to judge for yourself how you did in an interview, if you felt uneasy afterwards that may be an indication that it did not go well.

Application

How did you approach the application process? Did you treat it as one of the most important activities in your life? Were you professional? Did you apply early, follow instructions carefully, respond to requests from schools promptly, and treat admissions office staff with courtesy? Were your AMCAS application and any supplemental applications completed neatly and clearly? Remember that the approach that you took with these matters will certainly be perceived in your paperwork. While a neat, professional, well-timed application will not make up for a lack of strong academic and personal credentials, a sloppy and unprofessional one can be your undoing.

Consider the Alternatives

As you already know, getting into med school is not easy. Each year, many well-qualified applicants are denied admission. As mentioned earlier, the statistics for reapplicants are encouraging, with about one-third being admitted on their second attempt. Success rates fall off after the third and subsequent applications, although each year some of these applicants are admitted. Still, especially if you have been turned down more than once, it may be time to think about other options.

Begin by assessing your reasons for wanting a career in medicine. What drew you to the idea of becoming a physician? Was it a desire to help people? A love of science and problem solving? The intellectual challenge? Or something else? Knowing the answer to these questions can help you to start investigating other professions that may provide you with the same rewards and challenges. Do you want a career in the health professions or will another area, such as research or teaching, meet your needs?

Develop a Plan of Action

After you have sought feedback from the medical schools and your adviser, conducted a self-analysis, and considered the alternatives, you are ready to develop a plan of action. There is no magic formula. It stands to reason that medical schools will be looking at what you have done to strengthen your credentials for this application. By now, you should have a pretty good idea of your strengths and weaknesses as an applicant, and you should be ready to do what you can to improve your chances for success.

Remember to attack your weaknesses. If your grades are low, you can't fix that by doing research. If you have a GPA of 4.0 but low MCAT scores, you won't help yourself by taking more courses and getting A's. The same goes for other parts of your application. Remember that your personal and academic record were not made in one day, and it may take some time for you to show improvement. The following are some ways to improve your chances for admission:

Retake Courses

If your science grades were too low, or if the college you attended wasn't viewed as competitive enough, take harder or different science courses. If you got straight A's in night school at a community college, you may need to prove you can do the same concurrently at a four-year university. Even though it's a sacrifice to take a full-time course load, nothing proves you can handle the work of full-time science classes like taking full-time science classes.

Retake the MCAT

If you did poorly or at an average level on your MCAT, you need to decide whether to retake it or not. In trying to answer this question, ask yourself if you gave it everything you had to give. Did you take a prep course for the MCAT? Yes, we really do think you need to take one, and not just because we're in the business. Most people don't have the time, the resources, or the discipline to study on their own. Students who take a prep course benefit from the structure, study plan, instruction, and feedback that a

Alternative Life Plan

"I think it's important to have an alternative life plan when considering becoming a doctor. As a faculty member, I've seen many superb, well-qualified candidates who have not been accepted, and I don't know in some cases if I could tell you why one person got in over another. Keep in mind that the thing that you've chosen may not choose you."

—M.D., Johns Hopkins University, 1975

course provides. If you took a course and didn't like it, take a different one. If you did take a course, did you follow all of the advice given by your MCAT instructor, or did you pick and choose which advice to act upon? Did you study for several hours a day over four or five months? Or did you give it a few hours a day for four or five weeks?

Improving Your Chances

Some things you can do to improve your chances of acceptance the second time around:

- Retake courses

- Retake the MCAT

- Get involved in extracurricular activities

- Reconsider your timing

- Rethink your school selection

If you can *really* say you gave it your all, then you probably shouldn't retake the MCAT, even if you were disappointed with your scores, because your scores are probably "real." However, if you did *not* put in the time and energy into studying as hard as you should have (be honest, now), then it may be worth your while to retake it. Just remember that admissions committees don't give you points for perseverance, so if you're going to go through the effort of retaking the MCAT, make it count!

Get Involved

If you believe that your out of class record is weak, do something about it. Find an activity or two that interests you and get involved. Don't just observe, participate. Use the activity to help you to develop your interpersonal skills and ability to communicate. If you lack health care experience, now is the time to get some.

Reconsider Your Timing

If you applied late and interviewed in mid-spring, it's likely that your rejection was related to poor timing. Reapply the next chance you get, making sure everything is pristine and ready to go by June 1.

Rethink School Selection

It's also possible that you didn't get accepted because you applied to the wrong schools. Go over your list with your adviser to be sure you are applying to those schools that will look at your application in the most positive light.

Postbaccalaureate Programs

Postbaccalaureate programs are academic programs specifically designed to help applicants improve their chances of gaining admission to medical school. Individual admissions committees differ in the value they attribute to postbac work.

Types of Postbac Programs

There are three types of postbac programs, designed to meet the needs of three different types of applicants. The first type, which is geared for individuals making a career change, is discussed in detail in chapters 2 and 13.

The second type of program is designed to increase the number of underrepresented students (defined as African American, Mexican American, American Indian or Native Hawaiian, mainland Puerto Rican, and applicants who come from socioeconomically or educationally deprived backgrounds) currently entering the health professions. Many of these programs are designed for applicants who have applied unsuccessfully to medical school. Programs of this nature are generally funded by the state or federal government and range in length from several months to two years.

Unlike the other two types of postbac programs, the third type results in a graduate degree in the biological sciences. These programs are typically associated with a particular medical school. During these one-year programs, postbac students take classes alongside medical students, thereby giving future applicants the chance to "show their stuff." Typically, applicants from the postbac program are the first candidates to be considered for the upcoming medical school class by that particular medical school's admissions committee.

Is Postbac for You?

Whether or not a postbac program is right for you depends on which aspect of your application you need to strengthen. In general, postbac programs are designed to strengthen academic performance. Could you design a program yourself that would allow you to strengthen your academic preparation and performance? Maybe. But most would-be applicants do better with the structure and resources that a postbac program offers. Additionally, many postbac programs have feeder school relationships with particular medical schools. As a result, the most successful programs have acceptance rates approaching 90 percent. The downside of postbac programs is that many of them are located at private institutions, are

---

Pros and Cons of Postbac Programs

"In my opinion, there are a number of pros and cons to the postbac option:

Pros:

- You don't need any prior experience or preparation.

- You don't need to ditch your former life completely. Flexible course schedules allow you to work full or part time.

- Your fellow students will be more diverse, with greater life experience than typical undergraduates.

- Many programs claim that postbac students make exceptionally good med school candidates.

Cons:

- You may have to fork over big bucks.

- You'll have to work very hard.

- While your friends are working 9 to 5 jobs, you'll be stuck at home doing homework.

- You have to get good grades. Period."

—Postbac student, Columbia University

---

rather costly, and do not guarantee that you will receive an acceptance to medical school. Therefore, make your decision about whether or not to attend a postbac program only after you have realistically assessed what it can offer you.

Graduate School

Many med school applicants consider earning a graduate degree as a means of enhancing their medical school application. If you are considering graduate school because you believe that it will give you breadth and depth as an applicant, then graduate school may be right for you. If, however, you are hoping that your academic performance in graduate school will make you a more attractive candidate, think again. Many medical schools do not consider graduate school grades when they are reviewing an applicant's academic history. There are a couple of reasons for this.

First, when reviewing an applicant's GPA, admissions committees generally take into consideration the institution from which it was earned. Admissions committees know (as you do) that grading standards vary tremendously, and while they have a great deal of information on the relative difficulty of one undergraduate institution compared to the next, they have very little information on the relative difficulty of the numerous graduate programs throughout the country.

The second reason why many medical schools do not give great weight to graduate degrees is that a graduate education does not necessarily make a candidate more attractive. Assuming an applicant is planning a clinical career, the admissions committee will look to see that he or she is broadly educated, has the necessary interpersonal skills, and has demonstrated an aptitude for the sciences. It is not required, nor is it necessarily preferred, that a candidate have advanced studies in any particular area, much less the sciences.

There are a few exceptions to the above rule. As discussed above, there are a few medical schools that specifically use their graduate biological science programs as feeder schools into their medical school. These admissions committees will be particularly interested in applicants from their graduate programs. Also, if you are considering a Medical Scientist Training Program (MSTP), another M.D./Ph.D. program, or a career in academic or research medicine, graduate training in biology may be advantageous. Finally, there are some admissions committees that do consider graduate school grades in the evaluation process, and to the extent an applicant's record is strong, it will be viewed positively.

In summary, while there is nothing wrong with going to graduate school, you should not do so because you believe it will help you get into medical school. Rather, your decision should be based on the fact that you are fascinated by the subject matter, are considering it as a career option, or believe your graduate education will augment your medical education.

Foreign Medical Schools

An important distinction must be made between the 141 American and Canadian allopathic medical schools accredited by the Liaison Committee on Medical Education (LCME), and the remaining medical schools around the globe (foreign medical schools).

In general, we advise that you don't apply to foreign medical schools the first time around. Aside from the obvious barriers such as language and culture, the conventional wisdom is that the quality of instruction and resources available at foreign medical schools is inferior, although it certainly is possible to obtain an excellent education at one. These schools can vary wildly in quality since they don't need to adhere to any accreditation standard. In addition, graduates of foreign medical schools have a harder time passing licensing exams and gaining acceptance into residency programs in the United States. Furthermore, teaching hospitals are currently under pressure to reduce the number of residency spots. This means that it will likely be even more difficult for foreign med grads to earn spots in residency programs. You probably shouldn't consider a foreign medical school until you've been rejected from American or Canadian schools at least twice (if not three times). Then you should speak to your premed adviser and do extensive research on the quality of the schools that you are considering.

In summary, if you attend a foreign medical school, there is a real possibility that you will be unable to obtain a U.S. license (either because you fail the licensing exams or are unable to obtain a U.S. residency position). Therefore, you should only consider this route if it is all right with you that you may be ultimately limited to practice (and live) outside of the United States. If this is acceptable to you, then a foreign medical education may be a viable option. But if it's not, don't do it.

Osteopathic Medicine

Osteopathic medicine should not be thought of as a fallback position if you don't get into an allopathic medical school, because osteopathic physicians have all the rights, privileges, and responsibilities as allopathic physicians. However, some students do stumble on to their true calling in osteopathic medicine after being rejected from allopathic medical schools, as did the student featured in the sidebar on this page. This is an option that you also might want to consider.

For more information on applying to osteopathic medical schools, see chapter 4.

Turning Failure into Success

"I was rejected from most of the schools to which I applied. Osteopathy was an alternative path, and I decided that I wanted to try doing it. I have no regrets about going straight into osteopathic school rather than reapplying to allopathic schools the following year. Now I am where I wanted to be; I was heavily recruited when going through the process of choosing a residency."

—D.O., University of New England, 1995

Choosing Other Paths

As you think about your professional goals, you may decide that for whatever reason—length of study, financial strain, etcetera—medical school is not for you. There are a number of fields in health care that may suit your needs better. Here are a few closely related professions. In all of them, practitioners:

- Give primary and secondary care to patients
- Make diagnoses
- Have a decision-making role in the care of the patient
- Are well compensated

Physician's Assistant

Sixty-three U.S. schools offer Physician's Assistants programs. The programs average three years, ranging from 12 to 48 months. In many, clinical rotations are done side by side with third- and fourth-year medical students. PA's typically get their clinical training in many different locations based on which electives interest them. On completion of the program, PAs must pass the accreditation exam given by the National Commission on Certification of PAs to practice as "PA-C."

> ### *Less Pain, Pure Gain*
>
> "I realized I wanted to be doing primary care work, and I had no desire to spend seven years in school. I got out in three years and now I'm working at a women's health clinic doing exactly what I wanted."
>
> —Physician's assistant

PAs can act independently in a clinical setting under a physician, or they can bridge the gap in a hospital between the nurses and doctors. States differ on the degree to which PAs can prescribe medicine or sign for in-hospital treatments. Around 70 percent of PAs practice in a private practice setting, while 30 percent practice in hospitals.

Many students choose to become physician's assistants rather than physicians because of the shorter length of study and the less burdensome expense. Some realize that what they really want is to provide primary care, and aren't as concerned about commanding the prestige that doctors generally hold.

One potential downside of the profession is the somewhat limited choice that the PA faces after graduating. Generally, PAs choose a specialty during school, such as pediatric surgery or clinical gynecology, and will continue to specialize in that field after graduation.

Nurse Practitioner

Advanced practice nurses—nurse practitioners, midwives, and clinical specialists—have gained significant recognition and legislative practice authority as quality providers of primary health care, with a special emphasis on patient education. Nurse practitioners can act in approximately the same capacity as Physician's Assistants, although they must always act under an M.D. or D.O. when prescribing medicine. Nurse practitioners can function as primary care givers in both private practice offices and health clinics. There is always a connection with an M.D. in case the necessity arises to admit the patient to a hospital or to get a second opinion, but many patients may be entirely cared for by an NP.

Not for Women Only

Although fewer than 10 percent of nursing students today are male, more and more men are entering the field, often as a second career.

Nurse practitioners usually earn an M.S. or M.S.N. (Master of Science in Nursing) degree. Both degrees generally take two years of full-time study, but can usually be pursued part time. Many graduate nursing programs require the B.S.N. (Bachelor's of Science in Nursing) for entry, but an increasing number of programs admit students with other college degrees.

For more information on becoming a Nurse Practitioner, contact:

National Organization of Nurse Practitioner Faculties
1522 K Street, NW
Suite 702
Washington, D.C. 20005
(202) 289-8044
www.nonpf.com

Final Thoughts

There is another school of thought when it comes to advising the unsuccessful medical school applicant, which cautions against considering alternative careers in allied health. Adherents to this perspective urge applicants to consider the reasons they were attracted to medicine as a career. Do you like being in a position of authority and responsibility? Do you want respect within your community? Do you want to achieve a high standard of living? If these are the things that attracted you to the notion of becoming a physician, then you may not find a fulfilling, satisfying career in health care if you cannot become a physician. If, after careful consideration and some soul searching, you realize that some of the above motivations are yours, consider investigating other high-powered, intense, dynamic professions. Talk to your career counselor. Talk to family and friends. Pick up a book in the library or bookstore on making career choices based on your personality profile. Your ultimate goal should be to find a career that is well suited to you, whether or not it is in medicine.

PART FIVE

Special Considerations

CHAPTER 13

Nontraditional Applicants

by Cynthia Lewis

The majority of applicants to medical school apply directly after completing an undergraduate degree, typically in a science major. However, countless others take a less traditional route to the medical profession. Some people have an interest in becoming a physician when they are young, but for one or more reasons, do not pursue their interests. For other students, it may take years for their interest in medicine or for their self-confidence to develop.

If you are a "nontraditional" applicant, you're not alone. In recent years, more people from diverse backgrounds, often older people with rich life experiences, have been entering the medical profession. For the 1998–99 entering class, 26.1 percent of the 2,834 applicants who were at least 32 years old were accepted to medical school, which represents about 4.3 percent of all accepted applicants.

Who Are Nontraditional Applicants?

Nontraditional applicants often fall into the following categories:

Postbaccalaureate Students

Many students have earned degrees in areas that have not prepared them for medical school, such as the humanities or social sciences. These students are called postbaccalaureate students. Other postbaccalaureate students have completed their premedical course requirements, but have earned marginal grades in the sciences and need to strengthen their academic record.

Re-Entry Students

Some students never finished their undergraduate degrees, for a multitude of reasons, and they now need to complete their coursework in order to reach their goal of a career in medicine. For example, some women took several years to raise families, and deferred their own education; some people entered the military and deferred a career in medicine.

Career Changers

Some people apply to med school as the result of a career change. They may have entered a career in an effort to support a family, to meet expectations, or because the career was appealing at a certain stage in their lives. At some point in time, they may discover a repressed desire to pursue medicine, or they may even develop one after experiencing a family member's struggle with illness. Still others wish to change careers in order to make a more significant impact in the world. If you find yourself highly motivated to become a doctor for positive reasons—that is, not simply because you need a change from your present career—you may be on the right track.

You may fit into more than one of these above three categories, or your motivation for applying to medical school may be unique. Most medical schools do not single out nontraditional applicants. But, of course, your nontraditional qualities can shine in your application, so it is up to you, and perhaps a trusted adviser, to assess your strengths and to make certain that they are clearly seen and heard.

The Postbac Advantage

"If you enroll in a postbac program, you may have a greater chance of getting into med school. The jury is still out on this one, but postbac students stand out from the general crowd of undergraduates; they often have life experiences that explain their decision to go into medicine that make them stand apart from other applicants. Furthermore, admissions committees may feel that the extra effort postbac students put in reflects particularly strong drive and dedication."

—Postbac student, Columbia University

Preparing to Apply

Nontraditional applicants often ask what they need to do to prepare to apply to medical school. If you're trying to carve out a preparation plan, your first step should be an initial assessment of how much time you can devote to preparation, how supportive your immediate family is, and how much you have set aside in financial resources to develop your application. Rarely is it clear and easy to work out the appropriate strategy; you may find it helpful to share your background and concerns with someone who has worked with many nontraditional applicants, and to enlist his or her help to develop your personal strategy.

That said, below are some ways to prepare to apply:

Formal Postbaccalaureate Programs at Private Colleges

If you have a strong academic record in a nonscience degree and are changing careers, consider this sort of program. Generally, you will need to quit working and put full-time effort into being premedical in order to take this route. This may work best if you have ample funds and wish to complete preparation quickly. The benefits of this type of program are that you interact regularly with a small group of premedical peers, you will likely have access to an advising program, and you can complete your premed requirements in a compact one- or two-year academic sequence. MCAT preparation may or may not be included in the package. You may get more individual treatment in this type of program.

A few medical schools offer a subset of this program, where you would take courses with the school's medical students. You may earn a Master's degree upon completion of the program. If you earn top grades in competition with the medical students, you may have an edge in admissions at that school, or be offered a guaranteed interview or acceptance into that school's medical program.

> ### The Postbac Challenge
>
> "Postbac programs are especially tough for students that are a bit rusty. The attrition rates at many programs is quite high; the challenge of the material can be quite a shock and sometimes makes people remember why they never studied this stuff before . . . and why they shouldn't in the future.
>
> "Competition for medical school is stiff, and admissions committees know that postbac students do not have to balance the same kind of academic load undergraduates do. GPA for the classes taken in the postbac program, usually two years, is thus extremely important."
>
> —Postbac student, Columbia University

Inexpensive Postbaccalaureate Programs

Some private and public colleges offer free or inexpensive postbaccalaureate programs primarily for underrepresented minority students who need to improve their academic records. Some schools offer programs with one or two years of upper-division science courses such as molecular biology, embryology, and immunology, as well as clinical experience, research opportunity, and MCAT preparation. Eligibility requirements vary tremendously; some schools require that applicants have previously applied to, but not been accepted to, med school, while others have minimum GPA or MCAT scores. The duration of these programs varies, as does the cost of tuition and how much financial aid is provided. In addition, such programs may require that you reside in a particular state.

Informal Coursework

Like many nontraditional students, you may need to continue working full time, so taking premedical coursework at night or on weekends at a local college may be your only option. This route, though, has its drawbacks. Many allopathic medical schools view academic credentials from community colleges as less rigorous than those from four-year institutions. (Osteopathic schools seem not to distinguish between records from two-year and four-year colleges.) Some four-year colleges provide weekend or evening schedules to meet the needs of older, working students. However, extension courses are probably not the best way to prepare: Medical school admissions committees may have difficulty evaluating extension courses, and may not want to "take a chance" on someone who is an unknown quantity. Your best bet is to call the schools where you will apply to verify how they view these academic venues.

If you are going to take the premedical requirements on your own, you can do so as a second baccalaureate student (and you may be eligible to receive some financial aid). You may not need to complete that second degree in order to apply to medical school; you may just need some of the coursework from it. Or, you may register as an unclassified postbaccalaureate student, which means you can select exactly those courses that you need for your premedical requirements. The down side is that you may not be eligible to receive financial aid in this option. And, you may be totally without an adviser, which makes navigating the admissions process all the more difficult.

Grad Grade Boost

"I was absolutely amazed when I got into med school. My freshman year of undergraduate school had been academically poor, and I thought that it would be a major obstacle. But I think my dismal undergraduate performance was countered by how well I did during my graduate career in biomedical engineering and on my MCATs."

—Med student, University of California at Davis

Graduate School

If your undergraduate grades in the sciences were not strong, you may need at least two years of science coursework to prove to admissions committees that you can handle medical school, and to prepare yourself to do well on the MCAT exam. One way to do this coursework is to complete a graduate program. You'll need to assess exactly where your undergraduate weaknesses lie; it helps to have an adviser assist you. Then, select your degree in an area that will showcase your refined strength in previously weak areas. Suggestions include earning a master's degree in biology, applied life sciences such as ecology or molecular biology, exercise physiology, nutritional sciences, public health, chemistry, and so on. One important note: If you do not ultimately attend medical school, for whatever reason, make certain that this degree is one you enjoy and one upon which you can build another career.

How You'll be Assessed

Older applicants are expected to bring some interesting and fulfilling life experiences to the application table. From the perspective of admissions personnel, older applicants should have more insight, maturity, and self-knowledge than younger applicants. It's fairly certain that you'll be asked, "Why are you applying to medical school *now*?" Admissions folks expect you to have learned something from your earlier career(s) that may be applicable to your possible new career in medicine.

Generally, medical schools pool all applicants for screening and do not separate out nontraditional or older applicants. So, as long as you can reasonably and convincingly explain why you are applying to medical school now, your application stands a good chance.

Many older students wonder if age matters in the decision-making process. By law, medical schools cannot discriminate against you because of your age. While they can't outright ask your age, they can easily calculate it from your date of birth or high school graduation. Generally, students who apply by their mid-thirties stand an excellent chance if their applications are strong. You may have to be really exceptional for schools to consider you seriously if you apply in your forties or later, however. And there have been a few applicants in their fifties who have been accepted into medical school.

Acceptance Rates of Applicants by Age*

Age	Number of Applicants	Percent Applicants	Percent Accepted
20 and Under	361	0.9	71.7
21–23	19,892	48.5	51.6
24–27	13,767	33.6	34.8
28–31	4,150	10.1	31.8
32–34	1,199	2.9	31.3
35–37	752	1.8	25.1
38 and Over	883	2.2	20.0
Total	41,004	100.0	42.4

*1998–99 First-Year Class

Source: Medical School Admissions Requirements, 2000–2001

Academic Background

If you took few or no science courses as an undergraduate, you are not necessarily at a disadvantage. You'll need to start reviewing, taking, or retaking basic material, and then add other science courses in the required sequence. Most people take two years to complete the required sciences; some take three years, while a few can complete everything in one or one and a half years. Remember that having a non-science major may work to your advantage: Since only about 15 percent of all applicants are nonscience majors, your background may make you more interesting to admissions committees. Make sure you describe why you selected that major, and, if applicable, how you developed it into a career.

Undergraduate and Postbaccalaureate GPAs

Schools vary as to how they consider your undergrad and postbac GPAs. Some schools consider recent strong academic records (from postbaccalaureate and graduate work) coupled with strong MCAT scores a sufficient indication that you are a solid candidate. Others look at undergraduate coursework, usually in the sciences, the trend from year to year, and the MCAT scores; although they consider the postbac or graduate GPA, the latter may not outweigh poor undergraduate grades. Your best bet: Call the schools you are most interested in to hear how these factors are weighed.

Will You Be Taken Seriously?

Some nontraditional students fear that their career change will not be seen in a positive light. It's important that you tell your individual story—why you are switching careers, re-entering college after a long hiatus, etcetera—on your application and in your interview, so be prepared. Describe why you decided to go into the military, have children, or become a teacher. For example, "I joined the military directly out of high school because I was not sure I could handle college. I didn't have any role models in my family who attended college," or "My family expected that I would enter the family business when I graduated from high school." Then, explain why you would like to become a doctor now.

Medical schools want to know that you have clearly considered why you want to pursue a career in medicine. If you are a nontraditional applicant, this issue may be even more important. You'll need significant medical, community, service, and leadership experiences that substantiate your claim to your new career. If you have been developing these things for several years, then you already have a track record. If you have not taken opportunities to develop these aspects of your background, you must begin to do so now. It will take at least a year or longer to do this.

Get Help

"As a graduate student, I needed an adviser who understood how to assess my undergraduate and graduate record and to help me devise a good strategy. I needed a sounding board to verify that I was doing the appropriate activities and taking the correct courses, and that I was handling the application process to my best advantage."

—Medical student

Finding an Adviser

A premed adviser can help you plan the courses you need to take and the steps required to prepare for your medical school application. This may actually be the most important decision for a nontraditional student. You may be an expert in your present career, or have mastered the balancing act between family obligations and your work life up to now, but this is a whole new ball game—juggling family, college, work, and medical experience. A trusted adviser—someone who has experience working with nontraditional students—can help you set schedules and priorities, as well as find appropriate opportunities for you. Building an application strategy is as important as earning A's.

A premedical adviser who has worked with nontraditional students can also help you connect you to faculty mentors who understand the needs of nontraditional or postbac students.

Adjusting to College

If you've been out of college for a while, you may be daunted by the thought of returning, and wonder about how you'll adjust and how you'll be treated by other students and faculty members. One way to help is to join—or form—a postbaccalaureate support group. At one college, such a group has a monthly meeting at a cheap, local restaurant or at a student's home. Their stated purpose is to "address specific circumstances unique to nontraditional students; to unify, to become acquainted with peers, to provide an atmosphere of academic and social support; to share and build ties to the academic and professional community; and to increase awareness of opportunities that are related to our career plans." If your college does not have such a group, start one. Knowing that there are other students with similar goals and backgrounds can make the postbac experience more pleasant and rewarding.

The Juggling Act

Preparing for medical school is hard work, whether you're fresh out of college or have another career under your belt. But if you are trying to balance going to school full time, working part time, getting clinical experience, and spending time with your family, your task will become even more challenging. In fact, if you're juggling work, school, and family life, it will probably take you longer to complete the premedical course requirements than it will a full time college student. The goal here is to maintain the highest grades you can while keeping sane at home and still sleeping, eating, and having some social existence. Here, too, an adviser whose perspective lies outside of your narrow focus may be able to help you develop a reasonable schedule.

Admissions personnel will take into account that you are working full time while juggling part-time college and raising a family, but you must make this perfectly clear in your written application, secondary application, and interview. Make sure you explicitly state the number of hours per week you have been working, name the jobs you have had, and explain whom you are supporting.

Advantages of Being Nontraditional

Nontraditional applicants are often the most interesting premedical candidates because they have a broad perspective on life, as well as high levels of motivation and focus. Lawyers, corporate executives, engineers, and stock brokers don't wish to become doctors to gain prestige and large salaries. In fact, they will certainly lose earning power for many years, and may never earn as a doctor the level of their previous salary.

Usually, nontraditional applicants give careful consideration to their motivations before making a leap into another lifestyle or career. One student said, "I feel like one advantage I have being an older, re-entry student is that I really am certain about my desire to pursue a medical career. Moreover, I believe that I was able to convey this to most interviewers, which helped me tremendously."

For More Information

Medpath publishes a directory of postbaccalaureate programs and sponsors a national postbaccalaureate conference.

Medpath Program
Ohio State University College of Medicine
1178 Graves Hall
333 W. 10th Avenue
Columbus, OH 43210
(614) 292-3161
www.med.ohio-state.edu/colmed/medpath

Health Pathways, a newsletter of health professions career opportunities, publishes an annual postbaccalaureate listing each spring for programs throughout the country:

Health Pathways
Office of Statewide Health Planning and Development
1600 Ninth Street, Room 441
Sacramento, CA 95814
(916) 654-1730
http://www.oshpd.cahwnet.gov/pcrcd/professions/hpcop.htm

You can also contact the AAMC to get information on postbac programs.

CHAPTER 14

Underrepresented Minorities

by Will Ross, M.D.

At the 1996 annual meeting of the Association of American Medical Colleges (AAMC), the Association's president showed a picture of his 1965 residency class at Harvard University School of Medicine. They were all white men. Harvard's class reflected a time when *de facto* segregation restricted access to medical education for certain underrepresented minorities (URMs), defined as African Americans, Mexican Americans, mainland Puerto Ricans, and Native Americans.

Until recently, enrollment of underrepresented minorities in U.S. medical schools had increased steadily. The AAMC re-energized the national effort to boost minority medical school enrollment in 1991 with the launching of "Project 3000 by 2000," an effort to increase URM yearly matriculation to 3,000 students by the year 2000. In the early 1990s, URM enrollment continued to grow, increasing to the current level of 12 percent of medical students.

Yet the "diversity bridge" is sagging. In 1995, the University of California Board of Regents passed resolutions prohibiting the use of race or ethnicity as a criterion for admission to the UC system, a resolution that was later codified by voters of California as Proposition 209. And in 1996, the Fifth Circuit Court of Appeals, in an unprecedented reversal of the Baake Decision, rejected any consideration of race or ethnicity as a factor in admission to the University of Texas Law School, "even for the purpose of correcting perceived racial imbalances in the student body." After the U.S. Supreme Court refused to hear an appeal, the ruling became law in Texas, Mississippi, and Louisiana.

The year 1997 will be remembered as a particularly bad one for minority students seeking admission to medical school. None of the 196 African American students who applied to the University of California San Diego School of Medicine was accepted; the AAMC recently reported that the numbers of URM students applying to medical schools dropped 11.1 percent from 1996 to 1997 (in comparison to an 8.7 percent decline in white applicants). In states where race and ethnicity were prohibited from use in higher education admissions, the number of minority medical student applications dropped 17 percent. It's possible that the hostile climate created by recent rulings is discouraging minorities from even applying to medical school. And the number of minority students entering med school has correspondingly declined, from a peak of 2,014 in 1994, to a low of 1,770 in 1997. This number rebounded a little in 1998, when 1,872 minority students were admitted, but dropped to 1,732 in 1999.

Despite the legal deterrents to affirmative action, the need for minority medical student training continues to grow. Minority health providers have provided, and will likely continue to provide, disproportionately more care to the rapidly enlarging URM population in the United States (estimated to grow to 40 percent of the national population by the year 2035). Furthermore, URMs graduating from medical school are far more likely to serve in underserved areas than are their non-URM counterparts. Finally, a recent medical report concluded that African American physicians care for more patients with Medicaid, and Hispanic physicians care for more patients without health insurance, than non-URM physicians. For all these reasons, it is imperative that medical schools train more minority physicians to attend the health care needs of an increasingly diverse patient population.

High Diversity

Schools with a high percentage of underrepresented minority students:

- Howard University
- Louisiana State University
- Meharry Medical College
- Morehouse School of Medicine
- University of California, Los Angeles
- University of Illinois
- University of South Florida
- University of Texas, Galveston
- University of Texas, Houston

Choosing a School

While there are numerous factors to consider when deciding which schools to apply to, minority students often have unique concerns. According to one AAMC study, factors such as curriculum, financial aid, and the availability of minority programs and faculty mentors are of greater concern to underrepresented minority students than to nonminorities.

In the following chart, you'll find some of the issues many minority students consider in choosing medical schools.

Factors Minority Students Consider When Choosing a School

	URM	Non-URM
School Reputation	79%	77%
Curriculum	69.7%	53%
Residency Matching	62.4%	53%
Cost of School	61.7%	55.6%
Financial Aid	52.7%	29.7%
Minority Program	57%	3.5%
Faculty Mentors	55%	35%

Source: Fact and Figures VII, AAMC, 1993

Opportunities in Primary Care and Community Medicine

URM candidates are more likely to pursue schools that offer community-based learning experiences, family medicine clerkships, ambulatory and primary care opportunities, and classes in medical ethics. You can find out more about these programs and opportunities by looking at a school's published bulletins, talking with current medical students, and visiting the medical school's Web page.

Financial Aid

Financial aid is often the limiting factor affecting minority students' choice in medical schools. Over 84 percent of URMs, compared to approximately 50 percent of non-URMs, receive some type of grant or scholarship during medical school. Even with generous financial aid packages, 93 percent of URMs, compared to 81 percent of non-URMs, graduated with educational debt in 1996. There are minority merit scholarships available, as well as numerous loans, so speak to the school's financial aid officer. You might also inquire about programs that offer loan forgiveness for future practice in medically underserved areas. For more information on financial aid, including scholarships, grants, and loans, see chapters 19 and 20.

Programs for Minority Students

You can get a good sense of a school's attitude towards recruitment and retention of minority students by checking to see what minority programs they offer. These are typically sponsored by a school's diversity office, or office of minority or multicultural affairs. Special programs may include prematriculation programs offering review or refresher courses; mentoring programs in which students are paired with minority community physicians; board preparation courses; and academic assistance, including tutoring, skills development, and flexible curricula. Several schools have expanded summer programs that encompass academic enrichment, basic or clinical research, and clinical medicine exposure. These programs are usually offered to students throughout the educational pipeline, and often start in middle school or high school. You can find out more about programs like these by contacting the minority affairs office at the medical school, talking to your premed adviser, or contacting the AAMC.

Of particular interest are the Minority Medical Education Programs sponsored by the Robert Wood Johnson Foundation at a number of medical schools throughout the country. MMEP programs are designed to help promising minority students gain admission to med school. Since 1989, over 6,400 students have participated in MMEP programs; of those students who applied to medical school, nearly 62% have been accepted. Offered during the summer, the six-week program includes lab experience, clinical and research experience, academic enrichment, MCAT prep, and counseling in the school selection and application processes. The highly structured program includes mentoring by and M.D. or Ph.D. MMEP programs are open to students who have completed at least one year of college. For more information, contact:

MMEP
National Program Office
AAMC
2450 N Street, N.W.
Washington, D.C. 20037-0401
(202) 828-0401
E-mail: mmep@aamc.org
http://www.aamc.org/meded/minority/mmep/start.htm

In addition, most medical schools have active chapters of the Student National Medical Association (SNMA), a student branch of the National Medical Association, a prominent national organization of minority physicians and educators. The SNMA offers peer support, academic enrichment programs, and practical approaches to succeeding in med school. It also offers a Big Brother/Big Sister mentoring program for incoming students. As one medical student said, "The medical school experience can be grueling, but it's a lot less stressful when you share your experiences, good and bad, with your classmates. The important thing is not to try to do it alone."

Applying to Schools

Underrepresented minority students share many of the concerns faced by all medical school applicants throughout the entire application process. But there are a number of special concerns faced by URMs.

Self-Designation on the Application

On the AMCAS form, you are asked to designate your race/ethnicity. Most medical schools accept the designations at face value. However, once an applicant designates himself as an underrepresented minority, his application may be reviewed for the degree of cultural immersion or cultural identity with the specified ethnic group. Applicants may be asked specific questions about cultural identity during the interview. A complete lack of affiliation with the designated group may indicate frank dishonesty to an admissions officer—and dishonesty is not a good policy in any part of the application process—but it may also reveal assimilation into mainstream culture, which admissions officers tend to tolerate.

An increasing number of students identify themselves as biracial or multiracial on their applications, a designation that poses challenging questions to admissions committees, most of whom will assume that these students have maintained a cultural identity with the designated minority group, and are not using the designation for secondary gain.

The AMCAS application also asks whether you consider yourself to be a disadvantaged applicant. This is a difficult question to answer because, while medical schools have different definitions of disadvantage, they will try to consider the effects of disadvantage on an applicant's later performance. In general, if you feel that you were socially, economically, or educationally disadvantaged during your early years, you may want to consider answering yes to the question. If you do answer yes, be prepared to explain your reasons later in the admissions process.

Medical Minority Applicant Registry (Med-MAR)

As an underrepresented minority or financially disadvantaged student, you can participate in the Medical Minority Applicant Registry, or Med-MAR, by indicating your willingness to participate on your MCAT form. This free service provides your basic biographical information and MCAT scores to minority affairs and admissions offices of all U.S. medical schools. You will then receive information directly from medical schools and connect with the Minority Physicians Database. Registering with the Med-MAR can alert you to opportunities and help you find support from minority physicians who've been through the process.

Minority Candidates and the Application Process

Admissions committees do not have a separate process for minority candidates. While subcommittees may be convened to help screen applications, these subcommittees submit final arbitration to the full admissions committee. However, minority faculty members are commonly sought out to participate in and are an integral part of the admissions team. Minority faculty members lend a degree of sensitivity to the minority application through their common culture and shared experience.

Remember that it is essential that you submit your application early in the year. Don't wait until the last minute to apply. June or July is not too early. That will allow plenty of time for you to complete supplemental application materials requested by individual schools and give the admissions committee adequate time to review your file. Some medical schools begin interviewing applicants as early as October. Your file should be complete when the schools are ready to begin interviews.

Minority Score Cutoffs

Few admissions officers will offer statistics on minority MCAT and GPA scores. Disparities do exist between the scores of URM and non-URM matriculants, but it is not clear how much of the disparity may be due to academic preparedness and how much to any inherent bias in the MCAT exam and educational system. With all applicants, but especially with URMs, admissions officers consider qualities such as leadership ability, determination, compassion, maturity, and communication skills in assessing the candidates' suitability for med school and the practice of medicine. The goal of the admissions committee is to recognize the contribution that URM candidates bring to medical school by way of their varying personal experiences, and to interpret GPA and MCAT scores in concert with these personal, experiential traits.

The Medical School Experience

It goes without saying that getting into medical school is challenging. But excelling in med school is a challenge as well. For URM med students, medical school has its own hurdles. Minority students at predominantly white institutions need to take the time to bond with other minority classmates, and forge alliances with nonminority students as well. The most successful URM students are the ones who choose faculty mentors early. Having a strong support system of other minority students and faculty can help you deal with racially insensitive comments and overt racism, and can also make it easier to deal with any family or personal problems that may arise during your med school years.

Minority students have a huge amount to offer the field of medicine. In addition to being more willing to treat an underserved population, URMs and the socially disadvantaged may also provide a voice of humanism to the current debates on affirmative action and the delivery of health care to the medically underserved through their strong sense of empathy.

For More Information

You can contact the following organizations and publications for more information on minority student admissions to medical school.

The Journal for Minority Medical Students
203 Canal Street
New Orleans, LA 70119
(800) 661-3319
fax: (504) 488-7072

Minority Student Opportunities in U.S. Medical Schools (MSOUSMS)
Association of American Medical Colleges
Membership and Publication Orders
2450 N Street, N.W.
Washington, D.C. 20037-1126
http://www.aamc.org/meded/minority/minstud/msousms.htm

Minority Medical Education Program (MMEP)
National Program Office
Association of American Medical Colleges
2450 N Street, N.W.
Washington, D.C. 20037-0401
(202) 828-0401
E-mail: mmep@aamc.org
http://www.aamc.org/meded/minority/mmep/start.htm

Student National Medical Association
1012 Tenth Street, N.W.
Washington, D.C. 20001
(202) 371-1616
E-mail: snma@smart.net
http://www.snma.org/

CHAPTER 15

Women Students

by Cynthia Lewis

The numbers of women applicants and matriculants into medical school have been steadily increasing over the last thirty years. In 1970, women constituted only about seven percent of all practicing physicians. Now, the figure is closer to 20 percent. In 1999–2000, nearly 17,500 women applied to allopathic medical school, virtually equal percentages of men and women were accepted, and women made up about 44 percent of the entering class. Projections by the AAMC published in 1995 are that by the year 2010, 30 percent of the physician workforce will be female. Judging by these trends, it is a distinct possibility that before too long, the percentage of female physicians will reflect the fact that women make up over half the U. S. population.

While there is no such thing as a "typical" female medical student or applicant, there are certainly concerns that many women share. Women medical students often report they are concerned with gender bias, sexual harassment, societal expectations that they will be the primary child care provider, the need for adequate child care, and barriers to equal participation of women in some medical specialties and subspecialties.

Making the Commitment to Go

If you are a freshman, you might notice that there are about equal numbers of men and women who consider themselves to be premedical. By the time you apply as a junior or senior, 43 percent of applicants are women compared to 57 percent of men. Why the decline? Although there is no definitive answer to this question, women seem to drop out of the premedical pipeline when a crisis (academic, personal, financial, family, health) arises, and they are not as persistent as their male peers after surviving the crisis. Men seem to be hardier in this respect, taking the occasional setbacks or "failures" in stride, and

Vital Statistics

- Although more than 50 percent of the U.S. population is female, about 20 percent of currently practicing physicians are women.

- About 10,000 more men than women were enrolled in medical school in 1997.

- Since 1970, the number of female physicians has increased sixfold, from 25,401 to 157,387.

—Newsweek/Kaplan's *How to Choose a Career and Graduate School,* 1999

rebounding until they have no more strategies to try and "success" seems not to be possible. There may be an important message here for women: You need to seek a role model, a mentor, or an adviser who can nurture your potential to fruition. If your instincts say "give up," they may not represent a realistic appraisal of your potential. Check with a neutral source of information—not your uncle, the doctor, or your sister or your roommate, but someone who has a good perspective about what it takes to get into medical school. A trusted premedical adviser or faculty member may be that person for you.

Choosing a Medical School

While the reality is that most medical school applicants are happy to get accepted anywhere, you should nonetheless assess the characteristics that are most important to you in a school. What are some of the characteristics that women, in particular, look for in a medical school? What is important to you? Here are some considerations voiced by numerous women premedical students. (Of course, some of these reflect concerns of male students as well.)

- A school at which students help each other. One student said, "by helping each other we can learn more about different people and how they like to be treated."

- A school with an ethics elective and courses that focus on the art of dealing with people

- A school that provides clinical experience early in training

- A school at which the faculty take time to talk with students

- A school that offers childcare

You may also be concerned that women are adequately represented in the school of your choice. On the following page is a chart listing the schools with the greatest percentage of women students.

Medical Schools Enrolling 50% or More Women in Their 1998–99 Entering Class

Albany	Michigan State
Allegheny	Missouri—Kansas City
Brown	Morehouse
U.C. San Francisco	Mount Sinai
Chicago-Pritzker	New Mexico
Colorado	S.U.N.Y. Buffalo
Cornell	Puerto Rico
East Tennessee State	Rochester
Florida	Stanford
George Washington	Texas A&M
Louisville	University of Texas, Galveston
MCP Hahnemann	University of Texas, San Antonio
Mercer	University of Wisconsin
Miami	Washington University

Source: MSAR 2000–2001

Women as Medical School Applicants

As a woman, you probably share with many other female applicants some of the concerns regarding how you'll be viewed as a medical school candidate.

Many women are concerned that they will be taken less seriously than male applicants by admissions personnel. Administrators and physicians involved in the admissions process are routinely cautioned not to allow gender bias to influence admissions decisions, but that is not to say it does not exist. Older, very conservative men could be more likely to have these views (of course, older men are not necessarily biased).

One premedical student put it this way: "Throughout my undergraduate years, I never labeled myself as a female student. I have been surprised by comments such as, 'It's great that you are president of such and such group, especially because you are a woman.' Frankly, my concerns lie with the future of all physicians." This is probably the best attitude to have and to reflect as you go through the application process.

Women students also worry about being perceived as more emotional than men. It's pretty unlikely that you'll be seen that way simply based on your gender, unless you give the school or interviewer reason to believe this by some emotional outburst or other behavior inappropriate to any medical school applicant. For example, if you answer an interview question asking about your personal strengths by stating your empathy towards humans in stressful or painful situations, and you illustrate that statement with good examples in medical or nonmedical circumstances, that would not be taken as a "sign of being an emotional female."

Classism, not Sexism

"I've seen examples of sexism in medical school, and it's true that most of our instructors are male (especially in the basic sciences), but I've seen a lot of examples of really successful and accomplished women among my instructors, clinical preceptors, and classmates. I'm actually more concerned about classism than sexism—most of the students in my class come from upper-middle-class or wealthy backgrounds, and a lot of times they aren't aware of or sensitive to issues of poverty."

—Medical student, University of Washington

"Illegal" Questions in the Application Process

Medical schools know that questions about your relationships, personal or family history, or future plans for family are strictly illegal; such questions leave schools vulnerable to lawsuits based on sexual discrimination. You will never be asked such questions in writing on either the AMCAS or AACOMAS applications, nor on the secondary applications developed by individual medical schools. Nonetheless, there is the possibility that you will be asked inappropriate questions in an interview, and should consider how you might respond to them.

Is It Illegal?

The most common illegal questions that women are asked are about marriage, family, and childcare plans. Often they are questions that might be appropriate to ask in other situations, but are not relevant to your ability to study and practice medicine. If a question elicits information about your ability to function as a medical student or a medical professional regardless of your gender, it probably is reasonable; but if it does not, then it probably is not warranted.

You may be asked if you plan to marry, and how you plan to juggle marriage with a demanding career in medicine. You may be asked if you plan to have children; if you have revealed that you have children already, be prepared for questions about how you plan to care for them, and what your spouse thinks of your career choice. Some women have reported being asked rather outrageous questions, including those about birth control use, childcare plans, relationship issues, and adequacy of parenting skills.

How to Respond

First, try to answer the question in a way that is favorable to you without affecting your integrity. For example, if you are asked how you plan to care for your three children while you're in medical school, you can remind the interviewer that you have been successful in your past academic performance, and that you expect to continue to be successful in your future performance at their school.

> ### Women and Medicine
>
> The Council on Graduate Medical Education's recent *Fifth Report: Women and Medicine* delineates five findings related to women in the physician workforce:
>
> - The number of women in the professions is increasing
> - Women remain underrepresented among leaders in medicine
> - Women concentrate in a limited number of specialties
> - Physician gender has little impact on workforce forecasting
> - Barriers to women's equal status remain as obstacles to their advancement

Second, remember that you are not required to answer any question. You can point out to the interviewer that the question being asked is illegal. (However, you probably won't get accepted at that school if you do this blatantly or aggressively.) You could ask the interviewer how the issue in their question relates to your performance as a medical student, but you need do this in an upbeat and nonconfrontational manner if you wish the interviewer to back off and continue the interview.

As a rule, it is rarely to your benefit to offer information about your plans to get married and/or have a family, however tenuous these plans may be. However, there are situations in which you would want to discuss your personal life, such as if your spouse is applying to medical school at the same time you are, since you will likely want to attend the same school. It's appropriate to discuss with the school how they view both of you attending their school. It is a bit tricky, as rarely are both husband and wife perceived by a school to be at the same competitive level, but if you seek to attend the same school, you need to address this early with admissions personnel. If you are concerned about childcare or spouse or family support groups, don't voice your concerns to your interviewer; instead, check the school catalog, or contact the personnel in charge of these services to answer your specific questions.

Bear in mind that it is the rare interviewer who will ask an illegal question with malice intended, or with conscious awareness that he or she is wading into inappropriate territory. It's more likely that your interviewer is a physician who is accustomed to asking his or her patients scores of personal questions, and is not fully aware that he or she is "trespassing" in the particular context of the interview.

You can, and should, report to the admissions office before you leave campus any discriminatory behavior, illegal questions, inappropriate questions, or poor interview technique (for example, if the interviewer spent only fifteen minutes with you because he or she was late and had to leave early). You have the right to request another interview, and the school should provide it. If that means you must stay over another day, the school should help you with your arrangements.

Balancing Family with a Medical Career

It's not just medical students or physicians who find it difficult to juggle caring for a family and devoting time to a career: Since the lion's share of childrearing still falls on women in our society, women in all sorts of jobs and professions share similar concerns. However, female physicians and medical students have a particularly demanding professional load, and have specific concerns regarding the juggling act. Many, many women have managed to have both satisfying work and family lives; still, as a woman considering a medical career, you may have to make some difficult choices and compromises.

> ### *Goals of Some Women Premedical Students*
>
> - "To find a satisfying balance between the hard work involved in medicine and my personal interests and relationships."
> - "To find a spouse who is willing to accept a nontraditional relationship, and who understands and accepts my commitment to medicine."

Your spouse or partner may face days where you come home at odd hours, only to crash for a few hours. You may need to consider schools that provide adequate childcare, or flexible class schedules. Here's one example: A single-parent applicant with two children agonized over selecting a less expensive, public institution that provided a traditional curriculum during a forty-hour curricular week compared to a competitive and more expensive private institution that had flexible class hours, a problem-based curriculum, a small group setting, and early clinical experience. She selected the private institution because it allowed her to attend classes all morning, return home to two teenage sons in mid-afternoon, spend time with them at dinner, help them with their homework, and then to do her own homework in the evening. In short, she found a comfortable way to integrate her family life into her medical education with a minimum of stress. She was very happy with her choice. This student is completing a surgical residency now; she learned how to balance her family and medical training time requirements before entering a stressful residency.

The Single Parent as Applicant

If you are a single parent, you probably have particular concerns related to how you will be perceived, how you will juggle caring for your children and studying, as well as financial issues.

First of all, you needn't reveal that you are a single parent. Admissions personnel are not allowed to ask your marital status; even if it is revealed, admissions decisions are made without regard to it. The financial aid office will have your dependent information if you apply for grants, loans or scholarships, as most students do, but this should not be used in making admissions decisions. (If you find out that it *was* a consideration for denying you admission to a school, you might have a case for discrimination.)

As far as having time to spend with your children while you attend med school, there are and have been creative, loving, single mothers who attend medical school and become physicians. Yes, it is difficult; you may have to consider options that are less than perfect. For example, one older single parent with three children ranging from elementary to high school age let their father take them during her first year of medical school; later, the children moved back in with their mother. That mother told stories of how she supported her children under very difficult circumstances, sometimes not being able to come home at night to fix them meals, or to pick them up from school. She had to develop a support system in a city where she had no family other than her dependents. Yet, she survived this difficult situation.

A "Right Time" for Childbearing?

On entry to medical school, 6 percent of women and 7 percent of men have children; by graduation, 11 percent of women and 16 percent of men have at least one child. Most medical schools do not have formal policies dealing with parental leave; some are flexible, and others are not. Many schools allow a one-semester to one-year leave of absence for child bearing. Certainly, the case can be made that if students can take a leave of absence to do research, special clinical work in another country, earn an MPH or an MBA, why shouldn't they be able to take a leave of absence

> ### Some Common Concerns
>
> - Gender discrimination and harassment
> - How women are viewed in relationships
> - The question of marriage, pregnancy, and rearing children

to have children? With good planning and support, you can survive pregnancy and childbirth any time during medical school. Of course, it probably won't be easy, but the same can be said for the child-bearing and -rearing decisions made by any professional woman in just about any job.

The advice from women physicians who have had children during their training varies. Most suggest avoiding having children during the third year of medical school and the intern year, since these are the most time intensive and stressful training periods. To lessen stress, some women suggest planning pregnancies between the second and third year of medical school, during the fourth year when electives can be scheduled, during the last year of residency (not surgical), during a year off, or after residency.

One student said, "I plan to delay marriage and childbearing until after medical school, after or toward the end of residency." Another medical student had her first child between the second year (the last basic science year) and the third year (the first clinical year); her second child was born during the second year of her internal medicine residency, which was creatively split into six months on and six months off with another woman resident; her third child was born after she joined a group practice.

Here's another student's story: "I discovered I was pregnant the same day I received my first request to interview at a medical school on the opposite coast. The next three months were hectic, as I adjusted to my pregnancy, attended classes, and flew all over the country interviewing. The day I was accepted was one of the happiest and most fulfilling of my life . . . and so was finding out I was pregnant. Both events were planned and anticipated, but the inherent conflict represented therein is perhaps my area of greatest concern. One moment I am ecstatic and confident about the prospect of 'having it all' and the next, I am panic-stricken at the enormity of what lies ahead."

Clearly, there are many issues you need to take into consideration if you plan to have children during your training. Perhaps most important is that you need to have supportive family and friends to help you manage during this demanding time.

Choosing a Specialty

Some medical specialties are still male-dominated. Most medical schools and premedical advisors can, of course, tell you about specific cases of women who have entered surgical and other male-dominated specialties and have prospered. You may wish to spend time asking questions of these women pioneers to get a better idea of what trails you may be blazing, and whether those trails still beckon after you understand some of the trade-offs you may need to make.

Percentage of Women Residents and Fellows in Selected Specialties in 1997

Specialty	% of Women	Specialty	% of Women
Pediatrics	64	General Surgery	20
Obstetrics & Gynecology	63	Otolaryngology	18
Dermatology	50	Plastic Surgery	17
Child/Adolescent Psychology	52	Gastroenterology	15
Rheumatology	47	Cardiology	13
Child Neurology	45	Colon & Rectal Surgery	20
Neonatology	44	Pediatric Surgery	9
Psychiatry	45	Neurosurgery	9
Pathology	43	Vascular Surgery	8
Family Practice	45	Urology	10
Geriatrics	41	Orthopedic Surgery	7
Preventive Medicine	34	Thoracic Surgery	5

Source: JAMA 1998: 280: 836–37

Dealing with Sexual Harassment

In a recent survey, one-third of all medical school students reported being asked "illegal" questions during their medical school interviews; many of those asked such questions were women. But it is rare to find cases of sexual harassment during the admissions process. In medical school and residency, however, things change. Sexual harassment by patients, nurses, peers, residents and attending physicians is reported by more than 25 percent of female medical students and residents. Clearly, the critical mass of women in medicine has not yet been reached to inhibit this activity.

In Conclusion . . .

Women have an additional component of responsibility: They must be teachers and role models for younger men and women. Male physicians are required only to survive the initiation process; then they become part of the club. Has medicine changed? Most women physicians and medical students would probably say "yes, to some degree." As more women join the profession, perhaps we will reach equity in leadership roles for women in the professional organizations governing physicians; such equity can only help change some of the attitudes and unwritten rules that challenge women who seek to practice medicine.

For more information on women in medicine, contact:

American Medical Association
Women Physicians Congress
515 North State Street
Chicago, IL 60610
(312) 464-4392
http://www.ama-assn.org/wps

American Medical Women's Association
801 North Fairfax Street, Suite 400
Alexandria, VA 22314
(703) 838-0500
http://www.amwa-doc.org/

CHAPTER 16

Students with Disabilities

by Chris Rosa

Thanks to trail-blazing efforts of physicians with disabilities and the opportunities created by the Americans with Disabilities Act, people with disabilities are applying to medical schools in greater numbers than ever before. This chapter will attempt to guide students with disabilities through the unique constellation of factors that impacts their medical school decisions.

Are You Ready?

The access-enhancing mandates of the Americans with Disabilities Act, coupled with the promise of assistive technology to provide greater access to curriculum, offers people with disabilities greater opportunity than ever before to succeed in medical school. However, the decision to go to medical school and become a doctor involves committing to an intellectually, physically, and emotionally demanding course of study, including four years of rigorous medical school study and three to twelve years of equally demanding residency and fellowship. The decision involves a major commitment of time, financial resources, energy, and investment in the development of a professional sense of self. It is an enormous commitment for any individual, but especially for individuals with disabilities.

In choosing to go to medical school, people with disabilities not only commit the same personal resources that all students devote to the endeavor, they must also realign all of the access resources they rely on for independence. This reallocation of independent living resources to support study in medical school often significantly diminishes their quality of life in other domains.

If you are a candidate with disabilities and you are truly ready for a career in medicine, these sacrifices are surely worth it. However, in order to avoid regrettable decisions, you need to understand what it takes to be ready academically, logistically, physically, and emotionally for the rigors of medical school. You should then be willing to look at yourself critically and ask, "Am I really ready for this?"

Exploring the Limits of Reasonable Accommodations

Title II of the Americans with Disabilities Act guarantees curricular and programmatic access for individuals with disabilities in medical schools. The ADA requires that medical schools provide students with disabilities with the reasonable accommodations necessary for them to have equal access and opportunity to succeed in all aspects of the medical school experience. However, with this in mind, medical schools often require things of their students that may be difficult for some students with disabilities to accomplish, with or without reasonable accommodations. The current use of computers and other technologies in medical school instruction has certainly enhanced educational opportunities for students with physical disabilities; aspects of the curriculum that once could only be learned through physical manipulation can now be learned with the assistance of computer technologies.

While the development of these technologies has certainly improved didactic instruction, there remain critical aspects of clinical instruction that still must be performed physically by the physicians themselves. For example, a machine cannot teach someone to perform an abdominal or breast examination. In fact, physicians are legally required to know what certain medical conditions actually feel like tangibly when making diagnoses. Similarly, the voluminous amount of reading and memorization invariably required by medical schools may pose difficulties for students with learning and other cognitive disabilities. These demands are important considerations when individuals with disabilities assess whether or not they are willing and able to meet the rigors of medical school.

The Right Stuff: Getting In

Like all candidates for medical school, students with disabilities must meet the criteria for admission to the schools to which they apply. In constructing applicant profiles, people with disabilities should consider disability issues that will affect their presentation of self as candidates for admission.

Undergraduate Performance

Candidate performance in undergraduate courses is one of the most significant factors in medical school admissions. Because the medical school admissions process is so competitive, good grades, especially in the courses required for admission, are important to your chances of getting in. If your undergraduate performance was affected by a disability issue (for example, an undergraduate institution's failure to adequately meet your needs for reasonable accommodation, or a learning disability that went undiagnosed throughout most of a college career), you might consider using other aspects of your candidate profile—your personal statement, letters of reference, and/or admissions committee interviews—

to "explain away" a lower grade point average. While such disability-related explanations may improve your chances for admission, they often do so at the cost of disclosing your identity as a candidate with a disability.

To Tell or Not to Tell: Disclosing a Disability

While your personal statement, letters of reference, MCAT scores, and interviews with admissions committees offer you the opportunity to demonstrate the richness of your background and strengths as an applicant, these dimensions of the candidate profile are fraught with opportunities for others to learn about your status as a candidate with a disability. If you are concerned about disability disclosure, these aspects of your candidate profile must be carefully managed. The following are some tips to successfully handle disability disclosure in the admissions process:

- The decision of whether or not to disclose a disability in a personal statement is a very difficult, very personal one. This decision pits people's pride in their disability identity against their concerns that lingering cultural biases against those who disclose their disabilities to be perceived as somehow less viable by admissions committees.

- Speak to those providing you with letters of reference and let them know how you feel about disability disclosure so that they do not unwittingly disclose information that you're uncomfortable with in their reference letters.

- If you are concerned with the implications of disability disclosure, don't volunteer any information about your disability during admissions interviews. Asking a question like "Do you have a disability?" is illegal in most admissions contexts. However, if you are asked such an inappropriate question during an interview, asserting your Americans with Disabilities Act right to confidentiality will probably not help your admissions chances. Instead, consider simply and honestly informing the interviewer that you have a disability that, with the necessary reasonable accommodations, in no way limits your ability to be successful in medical school. Answering such questions openly and honestly may actually help your interview performance by demonstrating a level of maturity and comfort around disability and illness issues that sets you apart from your peers.

> ### When in Doubt . . .
>
> If you are at all concerned about disability disclosure, unless it is central to your personal statement's thesis or to your ability to explain a sub-par undergraduate performance, follow this general rule: When in doubt, leave it out!

Taking the MCAT Under Accommodative Conditions

The MCAT Program Office outlines a rather thorough process through which people with disabilities may request reasonable accommodations for the MCAT. In order to receive reasonable accommodations in the exam setting for the MCAT, a formal request for accommodations must be made to the MCAT Program Office no later than the registration receipt deadline. This formal request should be made as early as possible, since certain test centers may not be able to meet your accommodation needs; in addition, the MCAT Program Office may choose to consult with your physician or licensed professional to verify the nature of your accommodation needs. A formal request includes:

1. A letter from you that describes in detail your disability accommodation needs.

2. A letter, on office letterhead, from your physician or other specialist who is certified to diagnose and treat your disability. This letter should document:

   • A current professional diagnosis of your disability (no more than five years old)

   • The treatment provided

   • The last date of treatment or consultation

   • An explanation of the need for the requested accommodations

   • A detailed statement from you or documentation from an appropriate authority regarding any recent testing accommodations provided in the college or university setting

   If you have not received testing accommodations in the past, your letter should explain why you are requesting testing accommodations at this time (e.g., the nature of your disability has changed, there is a specific feature of the MCAT exam format that necessitates accommodation, etcetera).

3. If you require additional exam time, your letter should specify the exact amount of time needed and the disability-related basis for this request. Standard AAMC policy permits up to twice the normal testing time with the appropriate documentation.

4. For those with cognitive disabilities, documentation should include a neuropsychological or psychoeducational evaluation from a certified professional using reliable, valid, standardized, and age-appropriate tests. The diagnostician must provide a specific diagnosis and show evidence that alternative diagnoses can be ruled out.

Red Flag

If your score report shows that you took your MCAT exam under accommodative conditions, admissions committee members will be alerted to your disability status. If you do not wish to disclose your disability to them, beware of opting to take the test under these conditions.

It is important to consider that if your scores were earned under accommodative conditions, the fact that the exam was taken under accommodative conditions, not the specific accommodation given, will be noted in your score report. Scores reported in this manner may serve as a red flag to admissions committee members, alerting them to your disability status. Even though reasonable exam accommodations do not provide testers with disabilities a distinct advantage over standard exam takers, this distinction may cause even the highest MCAT scores to be considered less valid. Thus, if you are concerned about the issues of disability disclosure, you should weigh the potential costs of disclosing your disability to admissions committees against the potential benefits of taking the exam in the most accessible setting.

Your Premed Adviser: Friend or Foe?

While most premed advisers are generally supportive of otherwise qualified students with disabilities' medical school admissions efforts, a small number have been reluctant to support the candidacy of individuals with disabilities. With the number of medical school applications soaring, premed advisers are extremely busy and may attempt to dissuade individuals who are not perceived as viable candidates from applying. If premed advisers have preconceived notions about the viability of qualified individuals with disabilities as candidates for medical school, they may, knowingly or unwittingly, attempt to weed out people with disabilities from the applicant pool.

If you are otherwise qualified for admission, have realistically determined that you are able to meet the physical and intellectual demands of medical school, and are still getting resistance from your premed adviser, you may consider asking your college's Coordinator for Services for Students with Disabilities or ADA Compliance Officer to intervene on your behalf. Your alternative is to go it alone without the full support of your premed office.

Evaluating Medical Schools

Once you have taken the necessary steps to ensure that you are prepared for medical school and have sufficiently honed your candidate profile, you are ready of make a list of factors to consider when evaluating your fit with a medical school. Beside the factors covered in this book that pertain to all prospective medical school candidates, the following are some issues of particular relevance to candidates with disabilities.

Home or Away?

Limiting your choices of medical schools to those available locally offers medical students with disabilities the opportunity to draw upon the support of a familiar network of resources to meet the very rigorous demands of medical study. However, by limiting your choices in this manner, you may exclude yourself from programs in other regions that would represent a better fit for you academically and professionally. What's more, given the keen competition in the medical school admissions process, limiting your choices in any way may ultimately hurt your chances of getting into any medical school.

Sunbelt or Snowbelt?

There are distinctive benefits for people with disabilities to attend medical school in different regions of the country. For example, medical students have found that when they have moved to the northeast and midwest, they often enjoy a comparatively higher rate of disability benefits than those available in many southern and western states. They also often find that medical schools located in northeastern and midwestern cities are more likely to be located near accessible mass transit than many southern and western cities. However, medical schools in the northeast and midwest are also frequently situated in cold and snowy climates and on hilly terrain that tends to undermine access for individuals with physical disabilities. Schools in the south and west are more likely to have newer, more accessible facilities, are situated in places that are warm, flat, and dry, and are more likely to be near off-campus accessible housing units than those in the northeast and midwest.

Traditional or Problem-Based Curriculum?

Students with learning disabilities may find that the applied problem-based approach to learning makes the medical school curriculum much more accessible to them than traditional discipline-based or system-based learning approaches. Indeed, the problem-based curriculum's emphasis on collaborative learning among colleagues and self-study techniques is often much more amenable to the education of students with learning disabilities than the high-pressure atmosphere and didactic emphasis of the traditional approach. However, the drawback to choosing a school featuring the problem-based curriculum for students with learning disabilities is that they may need additional instruction and direction in study in order to pass the first part of the national boards.

Undergraduate Institutional Affiliation

Medical schools affiliated with undergraduate institutions offer medical students the advantage of utilizing these institutions' comparatively vast access-providing resources in order to gain equal access to all aspects of medical student life. These undergraduate institutions often have offices of services for students with disabilities that can assist in working out the logistics of curricular accommodations and reasonable academic adjustments, auxiliary aids and services (including personal assistance services and sign-language interpreter services), and accessible housing.

Assessing Accessibility

Once you've narrowed the field and have a short list of medical schools you're interested in, you'll have to make some tough choices. But before doing that, there's more work to be done. Here are the main factors to consider in judging how accessible your target schools are to people with disabilities.

Physical Access

The architectural and technological accessibility of medical schools should play a significant role in your evaluation of these programs. The following questions will help you to evaluate the physical accessibility of a school.

- What is the campus terrain like? Is it hilly or flat?

- What is the campus infrastructure like? Are walkways and roadways well-paved or littered with cracks and potholes?

- Are all the buildings related to the med school accessible to students with mobility-related disabilities? If not, what is the institution's policy regarding moving classes and other student activities to accessible sites to accommodate you?

- Are the medical school's laboratory facilities and technologies accessible to you?

- The school's medical library will play a central role in your medical education. How accessible are its facilities and services to students with disabilities?

- Are the assistive technologies that you need available and are the academic computing facilities accessible to students with disabilities?

- Just as important as the accessibility of the medical school and its curriculum is the accessibility of the teaching hospital where you'll be doing your clinical rotations. How accessible is it to people with disabilities? Is accessible mass-transportation available? Does the hospital have the necessary assistive technologies that you'll need to work there effectively?

Programmatic Access

For all students with disabilities, but particularly for students with learning, sensory, and psychiatric disabilities, the programmatic accessibility of medical schools will significantly affect your choice of schools. When assessing the programmatic access of medical schools and their programs, keep the following questions in mind:

- Most medical schools demand large volumes of assigned and unassigned reading. What are the institution's policies regarding the provision of reading and other course materials in accessible formats?

- What are the institution's policies on the provision of reader, notetaker, and sign-language interpreter services?

- What are the institution's policies on accommodative testing?

- Where does the institution keep confidential student disability documentation? It should not store such records in your medical school student files. This file is a quasiprofessional one to which faculty may have access; it is not appropriate for disability documentation to be kept in this file.

- Who has been designated by the medical school to provide reasonable accommodations to medical students with disabilities? In undergraduate institution-affiliated medical schools, is it the office of services for students with disabilities? Is it a member of the medical school's administration or a faculty member? The individual or entity responsible will serve as a key resource in students with disabilities' efforts to succeed in medical school.

Doctors with Disabilities: Peers or Patients?

Because of the impact of the Americans with Disabilities Act and the stereotype-shattering progress of doctors with disabilities, the medical profession has generally become more accepting of people with disabilities in its ranks. However, according to some doctors with disabilities, there are still significant pockets of resistance. According to one doctor, a physician with a disability confounds traditional roles of doctor and patient: He or she challenges some essential elements of the doctor-patient relationship. To some, doctors with disabilities look like patients; some physicians treat doctors with disabilities like patients rather than peers. This physician further suggests that this differential perception of doctors with disabilities is institutionalized within the medical profession through "Committees for Physicians with Physical Limitations" that exist in several states' medical boards, which serve to marginalize physicians with disabilities as a class. While not all doctors with disabilities share this perception, this cultural dimension is helpful in understanding some of the barriers candidates with disabilities may face.

Despite the obstacles that they may encounter, individuals with disabilities often bring unique insight to the role of physician. They offer first-hand experience of living with disability and illness, which may help them to build a better rapport with their patients and enable them to explain the implications of illness and medical interventions in very real terms.

Accessible Alternatives

While the physical demands of internal medicine may pose significant barriers to prospective physicians with disabilities, other areas of specialization may be more accessible to doctors with physical disabilities, such as radiology, psychiatry, pathology, microbiology, pharmacology, medical administration, and public health administration.

Lesbian and Gay Students

by Allen Maniker, M.D.

As a gay or lesbian person in medicine, there are many contributions that you can make in caring for the people of your community in particular or the population in general. Nonetheless, homophobia is a fact of life that you may encounter during your medical education and career. As much as you might view physicians as enlightened individuals, there still exist physicians and other health practitioners who disdain, or even hate, people with a sexual orientation different from their own. People with these prejudices may end up being your classmates, your teachers, or your patients.

Throughout the course of your medical education, as well as your career, you will be called upon to assess the source and target of any biases you encounter, and to find appropriate responses to them. In any given situation, you'll have to consider factors such as care of and consideration for your patients, damage to your career, compromise of your political standing, and insult to your sense of justice. You may feel so strongly offended that you are willing to pursue official redress for some comment or action, or you may just not feel like fighting on that day. The choices will not always be easy and each individual must decide for him or herself how to handle each particular situation—there are no right or wrong answers.

On the other hand, the gay and lesbian community has made enormous strides in the last fifteen years toward acceptance and understanding by the larger heterosexual community. You may be pleasantly surprised at the acceptance and the "nonevent" that coming out and being openly gay or lesbian may be, even in such traditionally conservative professions such as medicine. The advent of AIDS made the gay and lesbian community much more visible to the medical community, and subsequently reactions to homosexuals and their particular medical issues have changed significantly. Situations that you might have encountered in 1981 at the start of the AIDS epidemic are very different from those you might face now.

Gay-Friendly Schools

While there are medical schools that may be more "gay friendly" than others, it's not likely that you'll be able to identify them during the interview or overall admissions process. In large urban areas where familiarity with openly gay people is greater, you may find the environment more open, and therefore more comfortable. Centers with large gay populations, such as San Francisco or New York, will have even greater outreach to gay and lesbian students, though this is not certain. On the other hand, medical schools with religious affiliations may look less favorably on gay and lesbian students, although this, too,

Out or Not?

Unless you choose to talk about it, your sexual orientation should not be a topic of discussion during your med school interview.

is not a given. Yet whatever the location or affiliation, medical schools and academic medical institutions are comprised of so many people that the attitude toward gay and lesbian students might differ vastly from one part of the hospital or school to another. All in all, although being open with your fellow students and teachers is nice and even desirable during what will be a stressful period of your life, most gay students don't make finding a "gay friendly" school a major objective in their choice of schools.

The Interview

A school's policy towards sexual orientation in general, and your orientation in particular, should not come up during the interview process unless you as the applicant make it a topic of discussion. Whether you take a direct open approach or one that's more discreet is up to your personal views, and the "vibe" in the interview room. Unless you are very sure of your footing, the wisdom of bringing up your sexual orientation is questionable, since doing so risks alienating the interviewer. While taking a less confrontational approach or avoiding the issue completely may compromise your "out and proud" feelings, at the end of the day, the goal is to gain acceptance into medical school and become a physician. This should be your major focus during an admission interview.

There are approaches that can clue you in to a school's policies and attitudes without risking an unfavorable reaction from the interviewer. Before the interview, you should visit the school's Web site or ask for a student handbook regarding curriculum and policy. Then:

- Check to see if the school has a nondiscrimination policy, or provides domestic partner benefits.

- Find out if the school has a human sexuality program in the curriculum. One that does may be more committed to presenting a balanced picture of the range of human sexual expression, and may encourage tolerance.

- Take a walk around the campus and observe the other students and their surroundings. Do these look like students with whom you would want to spend time? Could you be comfortable with them in a working environment? Does the whole atmosphere of the institution make you comfortable? You may want to sit in on a class or two to see first hand the interactions between students, and between students and teachers.

One additional note: Although your preferred sense of fashion might be all the rage in Paris or Milan, it might not be appropriate for the admission interview. Physicians are generally conservative people, and this conservatism is reflected in their dress. As a rule, if you want to join the club it is probably best to look like most of the members, at least until you are able to get through the door.

The Medical School Experience

Once in medical school, your opportunities for being more open are greater and more in your control. At your school, there may be a group of gay and lesbian students who participate in an organization such as Lesbian, Gay, and Bisexual People in Medicine (LGBPM), which is sponsored by the American Medical Student Association. The Gay and Lesbian Medical Association (GLMA),which publishes *The Journal of the Gay and Lesbian Medical Association,* also has chapters at many medical schools. Organizations like this provide social life,support, and advocacy, but may maintain a very low profile. If there's no such organization at the

> ### *Help on the Web*
>
> - Gay and Lesbian Medical Association: www.glma.org
>
> - Lesbian, Gay, and Bisexual People in Medicine www.amsa.org/sc/lgbpm.html

school you'll be attending, you may want to consider forming one. The Office of Student Affairs in your school may be able to advise you in how to initiate such a group. Or contact:

Lesbian, Gay, and Bisexual People in Medicine Committee
American Medical Student Association
1902 Association Drive
Reston, VA 20191
(703) 620-6600
www.amsa.org/sc/lgbpm.html

Gay and Lesbian Medical Association
459 Fulton Street
Suite 107
San Francisco, CA 94102
www.glma.org

You'll also find in medical school that certain subspecialties may be more gay friendly than others. For example, psychiatry has a tradition of openness toward gay and lesbian people, while surgery and its subspecialties tend to be less accepting. Chalk it up to the "macho man" image of surgeons but nonetheless this intolerance persists and one should be prepared accordingly. Tolerance or intolerance by other physicians should not by any means deter you from pursuing any area of medicine.

While you're in med school, you may be subjected to homophobic comments, both overt and covert. Depending on the seriousness of the comment and the situation in which it is presented, you may choose to confront the offender, or educate or ignore him or her. Often, educating offenders is more fruitful than confronting them, since they might not even be aware that they've said something offensive. If a student or faculty member's comments begin to interfere with your work or education, you should consider taking official recourse, though the Dean of Student Affairs or ombudsperson, if such an office is present in your school.

It's more difficult to deal with homophobia on the part of patients. While it should rarely, if ever, become an issue, you should always maintain a professional attitude in dealing with patients and try to avoid confrontation. Many times a disease process may cause inappropriate behavior or dis-inhibition. Thus, an offensive comment may be a result of a disease process, so to confront a patient would not only be unproductive, but also inappropriate. Considering this, it's better just to walk away from an offensive patient. If you feel that taking care of a particular patient is really intolerable, you can always speak with your resident or faculty member and ask to be assigned to another patient. But remember that your patients' health concerns must remain the primary focus.

Residency and Beyond

Pursuing a specialty requires a residency position and therefore another round of interviews. As with medical school interviews, your approach to the interview must be individualized. Keep your eye on the goal of obtaining training in the specialty of your choice in a location or institution that you desire.

As you progress along the course of becoming a physician, the freedom you'll have for individual expression will become much greater. Once you are an attending physician or faculty member, your decisions regarding your openness about your sexual orientation will be more your own and less dictated by the fear of alienating someone else. Even though medicine is one of the most conservative professions, it is certainly possible to be "out and proud" and maintain a productive and fulfilling professional life. Becoming a physician entails a long, arduous, but ultimately very satisfying journey, and it is one that is most definitely inclusive of gay and lesbian people.

Financing Your Degree

CHAPTER 18

Figuring Out Costs

By almost anyone's standards, a medical school education is expensive: The total cost can exceed $130,000. The cost is high for a couple of reasons. First, the number of faculty members at medical schools is often two to three times the number of students. Second, faculty members command generous salaries from universities, which must compete with the incomes physicians would make in private practice. Third, schools must budget for state-of-the-art equipment and facilities to provide you with the quality of education you need to enter the field.

Though the costs of a medical education are daunting, don't despair. If you can demonstrate the determination it takes to make it past the hurdles of being admitted to medical school, financing your education should not stand in your way. Financial planning now will mean greater freedom to make choices about the many financial decisions that will follow medical school.

The first step in charting a financial path is knowing what all of the costs are. Only then can you develop a strategy for meeting them.

True Costs

Tuition and Fees

The most natural place to start assessing medical school costs is by looking at tuition and fees. Be aware that these will probably go up approximately five percent each year. If you're still an undergrad, you'll also need to factor the years until you graduate plus your four years in medical school when estimating the tuition and fee increases.

Tuition and fees vary widely from region to region, between public and private institutions. For example, at the public University of North Carolina, annual tuition/fees for in-state residents were only $3,353 in 1999–2000. But the University of Vermont, also public, tuition/fees for in-state residents were $19,777. For private schools, a student could pay as little as $17,898 annually at Howard University, or as much as $35,975 at Boston University.

Going Up . . .

Expect medical school tuition and fees to rise about five percent each year!

Public Schools and Residency

Public colleges are almost always less expensive if you are a resident of the state they are located in because the costs are partially subsidized by state tax revenue. However, attractive low rates for residents often mean that admissions standards are more competitive.

If you are a nonresident of the state, very often the added tuition will make your bill look much like that of most private schools. Out-of-state students at the low-cost University of North Carolina Medical School, for example, pay over $24,245 in tuition and fees. And out-of-state students at the University of Colorado School of Medicine pay a whopping $56,750 just for tuition and fees! That's nearly one and a half times higher than the most expensive private college.

Residency Requirements

While residency requirements vary from state to state, you may be able to gain residency status by living in the state for a year preceding your attendance at the school. But if you're planning to attend as a resident of a public institution outside your current state, make sure you check the residency requirements carefully. The time it takes to establish residency varies tremendously from state to state. In general, though, to establish residency you'll need to show evidence such as a state driver's license, a state voter's registration card, proof that you paid taxes in the state in the prior year, or even a utility bill that establishes the date you began living in the state. Check with the staff of the medical school itself or with your premed advisor for specifics.

The Budget

Tuition and fee costs are not the only consideration in the final price tag for medical school. Two other factors can make an institution with low or moderate tuition into a high-ticket item. In assessing total costs, you need to consider:

- Total budget
- How much scholarship, fellowship, and grant money you receive

What It Includes

Calculated by the school's financial aid office, the total budget includes all of the standard required costs associated with spending an academic year at the medical school. In addition to tuition and fees, the standard student budget may include costs of:

- Books and supplies
- Room and board
- Transportation (car maintenance costs or public transit)
- Miscellaneous personal expenses
- Equipment purchases
- Medical exams
- Licensing exams
- Curriculum-related travel

Budgets, like expenses, vary depending on your year in school. The budgets published by financial aid offices are well researched and based on real or surveyed costs. When financial aid administrators develop the budget, they have in mind creating one that is modest enough to prevent students from overborrowing, and yet adequate enough to recognize realistic required costs.

Two points are especially important to remember about the budget.

Average Costs

Most of the indirect (or discretionary) components of the budget such as living costs, transportation, and miscellaneous personal expenses are average costs based on the specific locale of the school and the particular costs of the students at that school. The concept of "average costs" in a budget is important for a number of reasons. First, it lets you know what a full year of costs are for the average student and gives you some guidelines for what to expect for expenses such as rent and food in that area. Second, if you are applying for financial aid, it restricts you to a maximum amount of money you may receive from all sources during an academic year. And third, because it is an average, it provides you with a benchmark against which to gauge and work your individual expenses.

Financial Aid Awards

The budget is a financial aid budget. It is constructed by the financial aid office, and is used to make financial aid awards. Whether you apply for aid or not, you can use these average costs to work out a budget from which you can estimate your monthly projected expenses.

What's Not in the Budget

Though the budget is created by each school's financial aid office, it is also governed by federal regulations. There are a number of items that the government does not allow a school to include.

Family Expenses

The budget can include only costs for the student, not for the student's spouse/partner or children. (It can, however, include child care expenses.)

Optional Equipment

The budget can't include equipment costs (for the purchase of a computer, let's say) unless the equipment is required for all medical students.

Car Purchase

Budgets can't be adjusted for the purchase of a car, even though a car may be required at some point in the program in order for you to travel to clerkships or internships.

Relocation

Unless you have the good fortune to attend a medical school in the place you currently live, you will have relocation expenses. Since expenses that are incurred before your actual enrollment can't be considered as educational expenses for the purpose of creating a financial aid budget, your moving costs will be completely your responsibility. Moving across the country can add thousands of dollars to your first-year expenses; these costs cannot be covered with financial aid.

Debt

Consumer indebtedness is another source of anguish for students who have lingering balances on credit cards from their premedical school lives. Consumer debts are often the most expensive debts around, especially from credit cards. If at all possible, pay off what you can before you start medical school.

Residency Interviews

Even though these interviews normally occur within the fourth year of your program, they are actually related to activity after your enrollment. This means that these costs cannot be included in a financial aid budget and must be planned for separately. (There are special loan programs administered outside the financial aid office that will provide funds for this expense.)

Beyond those kinds of specifics, aid administrators may also limit or expand budgets in particular ways based on their experience with students at your school. If, for example, your school is located in an urban area with good public transportation, the transportation component of your budget may be based on the assumption that you will use public transportation, which may be significantly less expensive than maintaining your own car. If the school has sufficient on-campus housing, the basic budget may assume that all students will live on campus.

In high-cost urban areas such as New York, Washington, D.C., Boston, San Francisco, and Los Angeles, the living component of your budget may assume you share housing if you're single.

Comparing Medical School Costs

Once you understand the basics of what costs are involved in medical school, you can start to make comparisons between what you will actually have to pay to attend particular schools.

Try to calculate what you may be allowed for monthly living and other nondirect costs at the medical schools you're considering. Subtract the tuition, fees, books and supplies from the total and divide by the number of months in the academic year (usually nine). This figure can help you estimate what the financial aid office may determine to be a modest monthly allowance for living while attending the school.

Next Steps: Calculating Aid

Once you've figured your costs, the next step is to determine how much funding a school may provide in scholarship and grant aid. The real issue is not the actual cost but how much you are going to have to pay. Although private medical schools may seem prohibitive because of hefty tuition charges, some private institutions have endowed awards in the form of grants, scholarships, and low interest loans. These awards offset their higher costs.

Some medical schools will publish the maximum amount of grant and scholarship funding in their financial aid handbook. Of course, your particular financial circumstances will determine the amount you're awarded. In chapters 19, 20, and 21, we'll detail the financial aid process as a whole, discuss eligibility for various programs, as well as how to apply for each.

CHAPTER 19

Applying for Financial Aid

Financial aid application procedures can vary more from school to school than the procedures for admissions. This chapter will outline the general application requirements and discuss some of the documentation required.

Get the Forms!

The first step: Get the admissions materials and read them thoroughly. Usually, general financial aid information appears in this application, including the financial aid deadline(s). These deadlines drive the rest of the process for you. The admissions application deadline may be earlier or later than the financial aid application deadline. In addition, sometimes there is more than one financial aid deadline. In the case of multiple financial aid deadlines, the first one may be for students interested in scholarship and fellowship assistance. A later deadline may be set for those students who are only interested in federal loans.

Key Materials

The most common financial aid application form is the Free Application for Federal Student Aid (FAFSA) form.

FAFSA

The FAFSA form is always required to request any federal financial aid. This form is used for "need analysis," the calculation of what you should be able to contribute towards the cost of your education.

The detailed financial information you provide on the FAFSA form is then run through a federal formula to arrive at a contribution figure. The calculations are explained in detail later in this chapter.

You may apply for federal financial aid using the FAFSA on the Web. To do so, go to the U.S. Department of Education website and follow the step-by-step directions. You may also apply for federal financial aid using a paper FAFSA.

If you were in school the year before you plan to attend medical school, and you applied for Federal financial aid, you'll automatically receive an electronic access code in the mail that will permit you to reapply for aid on the Web. All students may now file their FAFSA reapplication electronically. If this is not possible for you a paper FAFSA may be submitted.

Additional Forms

Many medical schools are not satisfied with the information you report on the FAFSA, especially when it comes to determining your eligibility for the school's own money. They want to know more about you and your family's financial situation, and they will ask you to fill out a separate application. Contact the school's financial aid office to determine if such a form is required.

Other required forms may include (but are not limited to):

- Separate school financial aid application
- Your prior year's IRS 1040 forms
- Divorced/separated parent statement
- Number of family members in college verification
- Scholarship and outside award documentation
- Federal verification form

Since some financial aid application deadlines are earlier than April 15, you may not have completed your federal tax form before the deadline. Most schools recommend that you estimate the numbers and then correct them once you get your taxes filed. Others want you to wait until you have all the actual numbers. Read the school's financial aid application, or check with its financial aid office to find out the policy about estimating tax figures.

Even though you should be careful on your financial aid application forms, don't work yourself into a panic about them. Mistakes happen, and financial aid officers don't expect you to be perfect. It's usually better to estimate a number than to miss a deadline while you're trying to verify it. You can always submit the actual figure to the financial aid officer when you have completed your tax form.

Forms: Round Two

Once you've submitted all the required forms, you may have to wait a while before anything else happens regarding your financial aid. The amount of waiting time will depend on the time of year the forms are submitted, the types of forms required and the specific application procedures at each medical school.

Meanwhile, the federal processor, a number-crunching center for the government, is crunching away on the information you provided on your FAFSA. Its calculations result in a determination of how much you will be expected to contribute toward your educational expenses for the upcoming school year. Depending upon how you submit and process your FAFSA, you may receive a Student Aid Report (SAR) in the mail. Follow instructions on the SAR or on the 'FAFSA on the web' site very carefully.

Remember, if you need money to attend school, it is just as important to stay on top of the process of applying for financial aid as it is to manage all the steps required for getting admitted.

Calculating Your Need

The calculation of how much a student (and family) can contribute towards medical school always seems the most incomprehensible part of the financial aid process. However, it is actually quite straight-forward once you know the guidelines and rules.

Basic Guidelines

The first concept to understand is financial need. Think of it as simple subtraction:

Cost of Attendance – Family Contribution = Financial Need

As we discussed previously, the cost of attendance is determined by the school and consists of the tuition and fees, room and board, books and supplies, transportation, and personal expenses. The family contribution is determined through use of a federal formula called Federal Methodology (FM). The FAFSA form that you file gives enough information to the federal processor to run your figures through this formula and produce a family contribution. The federal processor is a selected firm under U.S. government contract who uses the methodology approved by Congress to calculate your contribution.

> ### *Federal Methodology (FM)*
>
> A need analysis method developed by the U.S. Congress is used to calculate the Family Contribution (FC). The federal methodology determines eligibility for federal student aid programs.

Dependent or Independent?

For all programs that receive funding through the U.S. Department of Education, all medical students are considered independent. This means that your parents' financial information is not used in determining your FC and not used to determine your "need" for federal programs (even though the school may ask you to report your parents' data) offered by the U.S. Department of Education.

However, most of the programs that receive funding from the U.S. Department of Health and Human Services, and for many institutional funds, students are considered dependent. This means no matter how old you are or how many years it's been since your parents contributed to your support, or even whether or not you have a family of your own, your parents' income and asset information will be required to determine your FC and need for those programs. In some cases, even information about a natural parent who has been absent for most of your life, and/or your stepparents' financial data may be required.

Family Affairs

Federal programs for which you will be considered dependent:

- Exceptional Financial Need (EFN) Scholarships
- Financial Assistance for Disadvantaged Health Professions Students (FADHPS)
- Scholarships for Disadvantaged Students (SDS)
- Loans for Disadvantaged Students (LDS)
- Primary Care Loans (PCL)

Many medical schools do, however, allow students the option of not providing parental information on the application. At first blush, this may seem like a viable alternative, since the federal health profession programs are relatively small compared to federal Department of Education programs. But beware! Many medical schools award their institutional grant, scholarship, and low-interest loan funds based on both student and parent financial information. Before you opt for supplying just your own information as an independent student, find out what you'll be missing out on. For some schools, especially those in the highest price categories, institutional awards may be significant.

What's Considered

Some of the components reviewed in assessing family contribution include:

- Total family income from the previous calendar year (base year income)
- Net value of any assets (excluding home equity)
- Taxes paid (federal, state, and local)
- Asset protection for retirement
- Number of family members
- Number of family members in college at least half time
- Costs associated with two people working
- Income protection allowance (IPA) for basic living expenses

Before you start calculating, you need to understand the components listed above and why medical schools take them into consideration.

Base Year Income

The formula in Federal Methodology requires the use of the prior calendar year income to determine your contribution. This means that if you enroll in fall 2001, you will be asked to provide your calendar year 2000 income. For the majority of the population, the best predictor of current year income is prior year income.

Income Protection Allowance (IPA)

This allowance provides for basic living expenses not included in the standard student expense budget. It will vary according to the number of family members and the number in college at least half time.

> **Independence**
>
> Programs for which you are automatically considered independent:
>
> - Federal Stafford Loans
> - William T. Ford Direct Loans
> - Federal Perkins Loans
> - Federal Work-Study

Asset Protection Allowance

The formula includes an allowance for protection of assets depending on your age. This means that a portion of your assets will not be considered in the calculation because they are protected for your retirement. The older you are, the more your assets are protected.

Employment Allowance

The concept of an employment allowance grows from the realization that it costs to have both members of a married couple working outside the home. The formula allows for a deduction against your total income.

> **Home Alone**
>
> If you feel you may have compelling reasons to waive parental contribution, contact the aid administrator at your school.

Federal Methodology (FM)

The formula used in need analysis to determine an applicant's eligibility for most federal financial aid programs has been written into law by the U.S. Congress. Congress reviews this formula every several years and recommends changes to it. The federal formula was established to set objective standards that would be uniformly applied to all applicants.

Broadly, FM takes the income that is received by the members of the student's household, subtracts the taxes paid and the cost of maintaining the members of the family other than the student, adds in a portion of the assets, and then takes a percentage of the result to produce a family contribution. Although this formula may not take into account all aspects of an individual student's situation, it produces generally comparable data on all students applying for financial aid.

Application Results

Once the financial aid office has all the forms and data that they need, they may wait for the admissions decision before they review your application. During this waiting period, it's a good idea to check with the schools to make sure that everything is complete and ready for processing once the admissions decision has been made.

My Heart Was Set

A top med school and a lesser-known school may accept you. What do you do? Many applicants have their hearts set on going to top-flight schools, but accept offers from others that are more generous with their aid packages. Be prepared to weigh all offers based on many factors—including cost.

When the financial aid office finds out that you have been accepted, they'll make an offer of financial aid. This offer is called a financial aid package. The financial aid package can include scholarships and grants, a Federal Perkins Loan, a Federal Stafford or a Federal Direct Loan, and private loans.

Now you need to review the financial aid packages and decide where you'll attend school. Your choice may not be the school that offered you the largest scholarship. You need to weigh the merits of the financial aid package against the desirability of the school itself.

You need to look at more than just the amount of scholarship funds included in the financial aid package.

- What is your contribution expected to be?

- How much will you be expected to borrow?

- What kinds of loans are offered? Do they feature attractive rates and repayment terms?

- Will you have to work while you are attending school (if allowed by the school)?

These questions should be answered before you make your admissions decision.

Next Steps

In order to make an informed decision regarding the value of the financial aid package, you need to understand all the awards being offered. Chapters 20 and 21 will explain the various programs in detail, starting with "free" money—grants and scholarships.

CHAPTER 20

Finding Free Money

It's every student's dream: Getting "free money"—money you don't have to pay back—to pay for your medical school education. Free money can come from a variety of sources, including federal and state governments, schools themselves, and private donors.

Federal Funds

Both the United States Department of Education and the Department of Health and Human Services allocate funds yearly for medical education. For some programs, participating schools also contribute money. Eligibility for federal programs are based on financial need, as well as some other factors.

Scholarships for Disadvantaged Students (SDS)

Eligibility
This scholarship is awarded to full-time, financially needed students from disadvantaged backgrounds enrolled in health professions programs. For more information on the definitions of "financial need" and "disadvantaged" for this specific program, contact the financial aid office.

Award Amount
Scholarships may not exceed the cost of attendance. That is, tuition, reasonable educational expenses and reasonable living expenses.

Institutional Funds

Some medical schools to which you apply will have a pool of funding they call institutional grants or scholarships. While some of this funding may be reserved for awards made strictly on the basis of merit, for the most part this is the money schools direct toward students based on need in order to equalize grant and loan awards. Other than the small pot administered through the Department of Health and Human Services that is designated for students with need from disadvantaged backgrounds, these are the only "free money" types of aid the institution has discretion over awarding. And you can bet the aid office goes through some pretty amazing calculations to determine who receives these funds.

Eligibility

Some schools use grants or scholarships to reduce or "discount" the amount of tuition students with high need must pay. Others aim to provide a certain level of grant aid for all applicants. Still others award grants as a way of filling the gap after certain other types of aid are awarded. You can expect parental information will be required to determine eligibility for institutional grants and scholarships and that it will be evaluated carefully before awards are made from these funds.

Most medical schools also have scholarships that are awarded from endowed funds donated by an individual or organization and named for an individual. These are also free dollars. Often they are awarded based on the donor's eligibility criteria and can require some form of communication with the donor. The aid office will often let you know if any of these programs are appropriate for you.

Award Amount

Awards can range from hundreds to thousands of dollars. Each dollar you receive as a grant or scholarship from these sources could equal at least two dollars you won't have to repay to a loan program.

Scholarships for Service

Service awards are not exactly "free money": You've got to give back what you get, although not exactly in kind. These programs provide scholarships for students who are willing to practice for a given amount of time in an underserved area, with a particular population.

National Health Service Corps

The National Health Service Corps provides scholarships to individuals interested in practicing in primary care professions.

Eligibility

Priority for funds is given to prior NHSC scholarship recipients, to prior recipients of Exception Financial Need Scholarships, to students from rural backgrounds who want to return to practice in underserved rural areas, and to minorities who wish to practice medicine in underserved minority communities.

Award Amount

NHSC scholarships pay full tuition and fees plus a monthly stipend.

Terms and Penalties

Recipients are required to practice in federally designated Health Manpower Shortage Areas one year for each year of support they receive from NHSC. (The minimum service period is two years.)

NHSC Information

Every medical school financial aid office should have applications. The NHSC also has a loan repayment program for medical students who decide to practice at an approved NHSC Loan Repayment Service Site. Contact: National Health Service Corps Scholarship Program, Division of School and Loan Repayment, Room 7-22, Parklawn Building, 5600 Fishers Lane, Rockville, MD 20857.

Armed Forces Health Professions Scholarships

These programs require an application directly to the service branch of the Army, Navy, or Air Force.

Eligibility

While still in school, medical students are required to spend 45 days on active duty training in a hospital with pay, as well as housing and food allowances. Recipients are also required to serve one year of active duty as a medical officer (after completing his or her residency) for each year of program funding received. Three years of active duty service is the minimum required.

Award Amount

Scholarships pay tuition, fees, and medical insurance, as well as a monthly stipend. These scholarships also provide a reimbursement for books and equipment costs. Because the funding basically covers most educational costs, you may not qualify for other need-based aid. Since these programs are very competitive, if you're applying for an Armed Forces scholarship, you should also apply for financial aid as a contingency.

For More Information

Contact your local armed forces recruiter.

Army National Guard

The Medical Student Commissioning Program allows individuals enrolled in medical school to be commissioned as Second Lieutenants in the Medical Service Corps and to be transferred to the Medical Corps at the rank of Captain upon graduation.

Eligibility

Students selecting this option must participate in 16 hours of training per month and two weeks of annual training.

Award Amount

Students receive additional training income that could range from $2,800 to $6,000 per year.

For More Information

Contact your local Army Reserve recruiter.

Scholarships for Native Americans

These scholarships are available only for Native American and Native Alaskan students.

Eligibility

Recipient selection preference is given to applicants who provide documentation of tribal membership as children or grandchildren of tribal members. Scholarship recipients have a service obligation of two years minimum.

Award Amount

The Indian Health Service Scholarship Section provides tuition, fees, selected incidentals, tutorial services, equipment, and a monthly stipend.

For More Information

Contact the Indian Health Service Scholarship Program, 12300 Twin Brook Parkway, Suite 100, Rockville, MD 20852; or call (301) 443-6197. Website address: www.ihs.gov.

Private Donor Funding

There are private scholarships, fellowships, and grants for medical school funded by individuals, corporations, and civic or charitable organizations. Beyond being designated for medical students, these gifts are usually specific to the individual characteristics of the student. Eligibility may be based on:

- County of residence
- College attendance
- Ethnicity
- Gender
- Religious affiliation
- Practice specialty

Guidelines

Make sure you leave yourself with enough lead time (preferably a year in advance) to obtain applications and complete them by the published deadlines. Chances are good that you can probably find several scholarships that you have a good chance of being awarded. The trick is to manage the information gathering and application completion, since these scholarships don't have any coordinated deadlines.

Scholarship Search Services

You've probably seen ads for scholarship search services in your college or local newspaper. These services charge you a fee to access a database that contains the information also contained in those directories of grants and scholarships.

How They Work

The scholarship search service has you complete an application providing specific information about yourself, which they then feed into the database to find a match of potential scholarships based on your specific characteristics.

Search Service Scams

Many students who subscribe to scholarship search services are disappointed with the results. Often the services provide obvious sources. In addition, waiting for the results often means wasting valuable time you could have spent researching for yourself. Be wary of potentially fraudulent scholarship search services.

Resources on the Net

Surfing the Internet can be a convenient way of looking for money. Though you may have to spend lots of your time searching here, you won't have to shell out any bucks. Since Web sites are constantly being added and deleted, you may find new sites when you search.

Keep in mind that these "free" scholarship searches will be useful only if someone is putting up the money to maintain the database. And, perhaps more importantly, remember that you still have to apply for the funds. You may have 100 potential sources of private aid. For each, you'll probably have to complete a detailed application, and possibly write an essay. Before you actually spend the time applying, check to see that the award amount is commensurate with the time you have to put into applying.

A good site to check out is www.fastweb.com.

CHAPTER 21

Borrowing the Money

Student loans are an important source of support for medical students. Medical schools expect the majority of students with financial need to borrow at least part of their educational costs; you should research loan possibilities early in the aid application process. This chapter provides you with the information you need to decide which loan programs fit your particular situation.

It may take many weeks from the date you applied to receive the loan proceeds, so planning is essential. Also, since the rules and regulations for borrowing through each of these programs differ, you should read each section carefully.

Federal Loan Programs

The two federal loan programs available to medical students are generally considered the core loan programs, since they carry certain attractive features defined by law. These features include a low interest rate, low fees, and defined deferment provisions. The two programs are:

Huge Debt Loads

With tuition at big-name schools now approaching $30,000 a year, six-figure debt loads have become appallingly commonplace. For the 1999 graduating class, the average debt was over $90,000.

- Federal Stafford Student Loan Program (part of the Federal Family Education Loan Program)
- William D. Ford Federal Direct Student Loan Program

The terms of these two loan programs are similar. The eligibility criteria, interest rates, fees, grace period, deferment and cancellation provisions, and other terms are all basically the same. There are, however, some minor differences in the application process and certain repayment options.

The key difference lies in who provides the loan funds. The Federal Stafford Student Loan is part of the Federal Family Education Loan Program (FFELP), through which loans are made by a private lender (such as a bank, a savings and loan association, a credit union, or an insurance company) and are insured by a state or private guarantee agency sponsored by the federal government. Under the William D. Ford Federal Direct Student Loan Program, the federal government is the lender.

> **Taxing Details**
>
> Schools may require you to submit additional documentation such as your most recent federal tax form.

Most schools participate in the Stafford program, but only some participate in the Ford Direct program. The school you attend will determine which of these two loans you can apply for.

Eligibility for either of these programs is the same. You must:

- Be a citizen, permanent resident, or eligible noncitizen of the United States
- Be enrolled at least half time
- Be in good academic standing, making satisfactory progress toward the degree (as defined by the school)
- Not be in default of any previous loans without being in an approved repayment program
- Have progressed a class year since receiving your last Federal Stafford Loan (e.g., fourth-year undergrad to first-year med student)
- Show financial need based on the information provided on your FAFSA in order to qualify for the interest subsidy

Federal Stafford Student Loans

The Federal Stafford Student Loan Program provides two types of loans: subsidized and unsubsidized. The subsidized loans are a better deal, but you have to meet the government's financial need criteria. For either type of loan, you may defer payments of principal and interest until you graduate or drop below half-time enrollment. Depending on when you first borrowed, there's a grace period of six or nine months before you'll have to start repayment.

The Federal Stafford Loan Program evolved from the Guaranteed Student Loan Program (GSL) that you may have borrowed under in college. The concept of a federal loan program originated in 1965 with the Federally Insured Student Loan Program (FISL). The Federal Stafford Loan Program has the same purpose as these previous financial aid programs—to make loan funds available for students to attend post-secondary school—but the amounts available, interest rates, and deferment provisions have been modified.

Federal Subsidized Stafford Loans are available to all students who meet the "financial need" criteria. A federally mandated need analysis, based on information provided on the Free Application for Federal Student Aid (FAFSA), determines a student's Federal Subsidized Stafford Loan eligibility. Students who don't qualify for the subsidized loan or need to borrow beyond the limit of that loan can take out a Federal *Unsubsidized* Stafford Loan.

Borrowing Limits

Medical students may borrow up to their demonstrated need with a maximum of $8,500 per year in the Federal Subsidized Stafford Loan Program. The Federal Unsubsidized Stafford Loan Program allows an eligible student to borrow up to $38,500 per year, minus any Federal Subsidized Stafford Loan approved. The total cumulative maximum is $189,125 (including the Federal Subsidized Stafford Loan and all Stafford borrowing prior to entering medical school).

Interest Rate

As the program's name indicates, the federal government subsidizes the interest on the Federal Subsidized Stafford Loan. You're not required to repay these loans until after you leave school. If you have a Federal Unsubsidized Stafford Loan, you're responsible for the interest while you're in school, but most lenders will allow you to capitalize the interest, and not pay it until you leave school. Capitalization means that the interest accrues while you're still in school and is added to the principal at a predetermined time (often at the point of repayment). The interest rate on these loans may not exceed 8.25 percent. Applications and information about current interest rates and repayment schedules are available at participating lending institutions and on appropriate websites.

Fees

There is a loan guarantee fee and a loan origination fee associated with this program. They may vary from lender to lender. It is important to consult your lender and financial aid office for an explanation of these fees.

Sources of Federal Stafford Student Loans

Federal Stafford Student Loans are made through participating banks, savings and loan associations, credit unions, pension funds, and insurance companies.

Application Procedures

The process used to apply for a Federal Stafford Loan has changed significantly at many schools. What was once a paper process, has at many schools become automated. It is important to determine the specific process used at the school you will attend. Give yourself ample lead time so your

Name Changes

Federal Stafford Loans were formerly called Guaranteed Student Loans. Federal Perkins Loans were formerly called National Direct Student Loans.

loan funds arrive in time to satisfy the deadline for payment of tuition and fees. Even though the process in some schools is automated, it still may take a week or two to receive your funds. Paper driven, manual processes may take longer.

Promissory Notes

Terms of repayment are explained in your promissory note. Be sure that you understand them. Keep the promissory note; it's your contract with the lender.

Repayment

The amount of your monthly payment will depend on the total amount you borrowed, the number of months in the repayment schedule, the type of repayment schedule, and whether you elected to pay interest on the unsubsidized portion of the loan while in school. The maximum repayment period is usually ten years. You'll have a shorter repayment term if you borrow a small amount, since there's a minimum monthly installment of $50. Lenders are required to offer the option of standard, graduated, or income-sensitive repayment to new borrowers. A new borrower is defined as someone who has no outstanding balance on a Federal Stafford Loan on or after July 1, 1993.

If you don't meet the repayment terms of the loan, you'll go into default and the entire balance of the loan becomes due. If your loan goes into default, the lender may refuse to allow you to borrow again until the entire debt is satisfied. Check with your lender to explore repayment plan options. Lenders are trying to make it possible for you to keep in good standing with your repayments, and they're willing to work with you to help you manage your debt.

Deferments

Under certain circumstances you may be able to defer, that is, postpone, the payments of your Federal Stafford Loan. Deferments are not automatic; you must apply for them.

Forbearance

You can request forbearance in situations that aren't covered by normal deferments. Forbearance means the lender agrees to grant you a temporary suspension of payments, reduced payments, or an extension of the time for your payments.

Cancellations

You can get a portion of your loans canceled in special circumstances. Once again, read your promissory note for details.

William D. Ford Federal Direct Loan

The Ford Federal Direct Loan Program was authorized by the U.S. Congress in 1993. In this program, the federal government is the lender. Individual schools, rather than banks or other financial institutions, originate the loans. This program includes two types of loans: the Federal Direct Stafford/Ford Loan and the Federal Direct Unsubsidized Stafford/Ford Loan.

The eligibility criteria, borrowing limits, interest rate, fees, grace period, and deferment and cancellation provisions for this program are the same as for the Federal Stafford Loan Program. The Ford Federal Direct Loan Program has different application procedures and its own repayment options.

Application Procedures

The FAFSA and the other required documents that were discussed earlier must be completed. Usually, the Ford Federal Direct Loan will be offered as part of your financial aid package. Once you accept the loan as part of the package, the financial aid officer creates a Loan Origination Record, and electronically transmits it to the federal servicer for approval. The approval is transmitted back to the school, and the school produces a promissory note for you to sign. Once the promissory note is signed, the school can disburse the first portion of the loan to your student account. Any funds remaining after any unpaid balance you have with the university will be refunded to you. The entire process can take less than a week to complete from the point of loan certification to disbursement of the check. Depending on mailing time and the school's schedule for loan disbursements, it could take longer.

Repayment

Most of the conditions of repayment are the same as for the Federal Stafford Loan Program. Students who participate in the Ford Federal Direct Loan Program have three repayment options in addition to the standard: the extended repayment plan, the income contingent repayment plan, and the graduated repayment plan.

> **Don't Be Surprised**
>
> Procedures for the Ford Federal Direct Loan Program will vary a little from school to school.

Option 1: Extended Repayment

This option is similar to the standard repayment plan, but it allows the student to repay a fixed amount over a period longer than ten years.

Option 2: Income Contingent Repayment

You pay a percentage of your salary no matter how much you have borrowed. If you have a high debt, this option could require many more years of repayment than the standard ten years. As your salary increases, so would your loan repayments. The drawback to this option is that the longer you stay in repayment, the more interest you pay on the loan. Indeed, if your payment does not cover current interest due, unpaid interest will be capitalized, increasing the amount of principal you owe.

Option 3: Graduated Repayment

This allows you to opt for lower payments at the beginning of the repayment cycle when your salary is lower. The payments automatically increase as the years progress. The repayment term may be extended beyond 10 years but the payments are more manageable in the beginning when you probably have a lower salary.

No matter what repayment option you select, the plan will be explained in the promissory note you sign. Repayments will be made to a federal loan servicer contracted by the U.S. Department of Education.

Federal Perkins Student Loan

> ### Maybe/Maybe Not
>
> Not all schools allocate Federal Perkins Loan funds to graduate and professional students.

Administered by colleges and universities, the Federal Perkins Student Loan Program is made possible through a combination of resources: an annual allocation from the U.S. Department of Education, a contribution from the participating educational institution, and repayments by previous borrowers. The program was originally called the National Defense Student Loan Program when it was instituted by the federal government more than 30 years ago. The program was one of the first financial aid programs instituted by the federal government.

Eligibility

The school determines eligibility for Federal Perkins Loans based on your financial need (calculated through the FAFSA) and the availability of funds. Besides demonstrating financial need, you have to be enrolled at least half time and maintain satisfactory progress toward a degree. Keep in mind that Federal Perkins Loans are reserved for the neediest students.

Borrowing Limits

Federal policy allows a maximum annual loan of $6,000 per graduate-level student. However, many schools lack the funds to allocate this much to any one student. A graduate student may borrow up to a cumulative total of $40,000, including all outstanding undergraduate and graduate Federal Perkins Loans.

Interest Rate

The terms are very good. The annual interest rate is currently five percent. Interest does not accrue while the borrower remains enrolled at least half time.

Fees

Another perk of the Federal Perkins Loan Program: no fees.

Application Procedures

Usually, you're automatically considered for this loan when you apply for financial aid. If you've been offered and have accepted a Federal Perkins Loan, you'll sign a promissory note. The promissory note lists the amount of the loan and states your rights and responsibilities as a borrower. When the signed note is received, either your account will be credited for one semester's portion of the loan, or a check will be cut for you directly.

Grace Period

Federal Perkins Loans have a six-month grace period after you graduate or drop below half-time attendance. During this period no repayment is required and no interest accrues. If you borrowed under the NDSL Program, you may have a different grace period. You need to check with the school that granted you the loan to find out the grace period for your particular loan.

Repayment

Borrowers under the Federal Perkins Loan program repay the school, although there may be a middle man: Many schools contract with outside agencies for billing and collection. Repayment may extend up to 10 years, beginning six months (your grace period) after you cease to be enrolled at least half time. The amount of the monthly payment and the maximum number of months allowed for repayment is based on the total amount borrowed. The federal government has set the minimum monthly payment at $40. Under some special circumstances, borrowers may make arrangements to repay a lower amount or to extend the repayment period. There is no prepayment penalty.

Deferments

You can defer payments of your Federal Perkins Loan until you graduate or drop below half time. This deferment is not automatic; you must request the deferment forms from either your school or from the billing agency where you are repaying the loan.

Cancellations

This might not make you jump for joy, but it's good to know. The entirety of your Federal Perkins Loans and/or NDSLs will be canceled if you become permanently disabled—or die. You can get a portion of your loans canceled in less drastic circumstances, if you:

- Teach handicapped children
- Teach in a designated elementary or secondary school that serves low-income students
- Work in a specified Head Start program or serve as a VISTA or Peace Corps volunteer

Check your promissory note. Your loan may have additional cancellation provisions. Also, if you have "old" Federal Perkins, there may be some different conditions depending on when the original loan was made. Check with your previous school for any special circumstances.

Federal Loan Consolidation

Federal Loan Consolidation allows students with substantial debt to combine several federal loans into one larger loan with a longer repayment schedule. The new loan has an interest rate based on the weighted average of the rates of the consolidated loans and may not exceed 8.25%. Stafford Loans, Federal Insured Student Loans (FISLs), Federal Perkins Loans, PLUS loans to students, parent PLUS Loans made after 1986, SLS, Health Professions Student Loans, Health Education Assistance Loans, and Nursing Student Loan Program loans may be consolidated only by lenders that have an agreement with the Department or a guaranty agency for that purpose.

To qualify for federal loan consolidation, you must be in the grace period or in repayment status on all loans being consolidated; if in default, you must have made satisfactory arrangements to repay the defaulted loan. To consolidate a defaulted loan, you must make three consecutive reasonable and affordable monthly payments. A borrower in default can qualify for a Federal Consolidation Loan without having to make three required payments if the borrower agrees to repay the loan under the income-sensitive repayment plan.

Furthermore, a borrower in default must not have another consolidation loan application pending; must agree to notify the loan holder of any address changes; and must certify that the lender holds the borrower's outstanding loan that is being consolidated or that the borrower has unsuccessfully sought a loan from the holders of the outstanding loans and was unable to secure a Consolidation Loan from the holder.

If you are unable to obtain a Federal Consolidation Loan from a lender eligible to make such loans, you may apply through the U.S. Department of Education for a Federal Direct Consolidation loan. You must certify that you have been unable to obtain from an eligible lender a Federal Consolidation Loan, or a Federal Consolidation Loan with income-sensitive repayment terms acceptable to the borrower.

You have the option of consolidating all eligible loans or only some of your loans. Often, students consolidate their higher interest loans, but keep their Federal Perkins Loans separate since the interest rate is so low. No fees are charged to participate in this program.

If you consolidate your loans you have the option of choosing the most appropriate repayment plan for you and your circumstances. These options include level repayment, graduated repayment or income-sensitive repayment. You should consult one of the websites noted at the end of this chapter for detailed information on loan consolidation.

For Medical Students

The federal Department of Health and Human Services has a few loan programs designed specifically for students in certain health professions. Contact your school's financial aid office to determine if they participate in the loan programs that follow.

Loans for Disadvantaged Students (LDS)

Funds for this low-interest loan program are directed toward students who have exceptional need and come from disadvantaged backgrounds. Interest on the loan is five percent and begins to accrue nine months after the month you complete medical school. Annual awards may not exceed tuition plus $2,500. LDS does not have a primary care practice requirement. For more information, contact your school's financial aid office.

Primary Care Loans (PCL)

These low-interest loans are specifically for students intending to practice in a primary care field. Interest on the loans is five percent, beginning nine months after the month you complete medical school. Maximum loans are made up to the amount of tuition plus $2,500 in combination with LDS.

If you receive a Primary Care Loan and agree to select a primary care residency and practice in a primary care specialty until the loan is paid in full, you pay only five percent. But if you do not complete your agreement, your five percent interest will rise to 12 percent and will be recalculated from the time the loan was made until it is completely repaid. That's a pretty stiff penalty, so when taking out this loan, be prepared to meet your commitment.

Defaulting on Loans

Defaulting health professionals received a lot of negative press several years ago. This led the Department of Health and Human Services to beef up the measures it takes when a borrower defaults on an HHS loan. Now, if you default on an HHS loan, it may:

- Report you to one or more credit reporting agencies if your payment is just 60 days past due
- Obtain a judgment placing a lien against your assets
- Assign your defaulted loans to the Department of Justice for collection
- Offset any IRS tax refund you might receive
- Publish your name, address, and amount of loans in default in the Federal Register (which invariably makes it to your hometown newspaper)
- Release information about your default to "other interested organizations" including professional and specialty organizations, hospitals, and state licensing boards
- Exclude you from Medicare and Medicaid reimbursement

Clearly, you don't want to default on any educational loan. There are simply too many ugly things that happen if you do. There are also a number of loan forgiveness programs and other options that make repayment easier if you've hit a snag.

Loan Repayment Forgiveness Programs

There are several loan programs under which you promise to put in a certain amount of time in exchange for reduced levels of debt. While they require a significant time commitment, they can reduce the size of your educational debt tremendously.

National Health Service Corps Loan Repayment

Program Physicians may receive repayment of health professions loans up to $35,000 annually in exchange for serving full time at a designated NHSC site. Participants are also reimbursed for increased federal, state, and local income taxes resulting from the loan repayment. Service commitments range from two to four years; priority for selection is given to doctors who have completed their residencies in fields of need at the time of application.

Indian Health Service Loan Repayment Program

Participants are paid up to $25,000 per year toward loan repayment for each year of full-time clinical practice at a designated IHS location. Priority is given to physicians in specialties of need as determined by the IHS.

Department of Defense Financial Assistance Program

Participants receive a commission in the Medical Corps of the Reserves on inactive status while in residency or fellowship, an annual grant of approximately $15,000, a monthly stipend of approximately $800 while in residency, payment of all educational expenses while in school, and an appointment in the Medical Corps Reserves on an active basis at the completion of the residency or fellowship program. The active duty obligation is two years for the first year of participation as a resident or fellow, plus one half year for each additional half year of participation. An eight-year Reserve commission that can be served on inactive status is also required.

Private Loan Programs

Many medical students find that scholarship funds offered and the federal loan programs are not adequate to meet expenses in a full-time program. Over the last few years, several private loan programs have emerged to fill the gap.

As the economic environment changes, new private loan programs are added and some older programs are discontinued. Check with the individual programs for their current provisions.

The Kaplan/American Express Student Loan Program

Through the Kaplan/American Express™ Student Loan Program, students can get information and advice about how to meet the cost of medical school. Kaplan/American Express directs you to the financing you need to reach your educational goals.

Why Kaplan/American Express? Information and guidance is provided through seminars, and written material. Additional benefits include:

- Student loan experts who are available to answer questions seven days a week, twelve hours a day, at 1-888-527-5626.
- Application editing by Kaplan/American Express experts who will review all entries, signatures, and figures on your application thoroughly to ensure accuracy and eliminate certification delays due to missing information.
- The Second Review℠, Kaplan/American Express's credit re-evaluation program, which guides previously denied borrowers through the process of clearing incorrect and/or outdated credit report listings and, if possible, reverses a credit-denied status.

AAMC MEDLOANS Alternative Loan Program

Sponsored by the Association of American Medical Colleges, this program is intended to provide med students with educational loans and loan consolidation services at competitive rates, as well as term life insurance and loans covering expenses related to residency interview travel.

There are numerous other private alternative loan programs. Contact your financial aid officer for information on private loan programs such as MedCap, Access, MedFunds, TERI, Grad EXCEL, and T.H.E.

Debt Management

You've read the material on financial aid and loans. You've done the worksheets about paying for your medical degree. How much did you calculate you'd need to borrow? This is the time to figure out if you'll actually be able to manage your projected debt. If your projected indebtedness seems unmanageable, now is the time to try to figure out ways to reduce your borrowing.

Step One: Calculate Your Monthly Payments

Use the worksheet at the end of this chapter to calculate your monthly repayments after graduating. In estimating your indebtedness, remember that you're likely to need similar funding for all four years you're in med school. Multiply all the loan amounts in your financial aid award letter by four to arrive at the total amount.

Monthly Loan Payments*

For a $1,000 Loan

Rate	60 Months	120 Months	180 Months	240 Months	300 Months
5%	$18.87	$10.61	$7.91	$6.60	$5.85
6%	19.33	11.10	8.44	7.16	6.44
7%	19.80	11.61	8.99	7.75	7.07
8%	20.28	12.13	9,56	8.36	7.72
9%	20.76	12.67	10.14	9.00	8.39
10%	21.25	13.22	10.75	9.65	9.09
11%	21.74	13.77	11.37	10.32	9.80
12%	22.24	14.35	12.00	11.01	10.53
13%	22.75	14.93	12.65	11.72	11.28
14%	23.27	15.53	13.32	12.44	12.04
16%	24.32	16.75	14.69	13.91	13.59
18%	25.39	18.02	16.10	15.43	15.17
20%	26.49	19.33	17.56	16.99	16.78

* Minimum monthly payment may apply regardless of the loan amount.

Use the table above to help you calculate most monthly payments on a level-payment plan over five to 30 years. For example, suppose you had a $5,000 loan at eight percent interest and a ten-year payment term. As the table shows, the monthly payment for a $1,000 loan would be $12.13. Multiply this by five to get $60.65.

Bear in mind, however, that you may need to calculate several payments. Each lender, under each loan program, should be calculated separately. For example, if you have several Federal Stafford Student Loans issued by a single lender, add them up to arrive at a single balance. But, if you have two additional loans issued under a private supplemental loan program, consider them separately. Calculate the separate payments, then add them together to determine your total payment responsibility.

Step Two: Estimate Your Starting Salary

Most resident starting salaries are around $30,000, and average salaries will increase as your medical career commences. Try to get more specific information from your school's financial aid office about salaries for particular specialties and types of practices you're considering.

Step Three: Fill Out the "Will My Paycheck Cover My Expenses?" Worksheet

The worksheet at the end of this chapter is very important. It'll help you find out whether your projected post-school paycheck will cover all your expenses. Many of the expenses in this chart are flexible. It'll be up to you to stretch your salary to meet your projected expenses.

Step Four: Consider Your Financial Options

After doing the "Will My Paycheck Cover My Expenses?" worksheet, you'll have a better idea of your postmed school financial picture. If things look tight, you could plan to reduce items in the "Discretionary Expenses" category. Another option is to lower your monthly loan payments. If you wish to adjust your loan payments rather than your living expenses, you must do so now rather than when you graduate. Potential employers won't increase your starting salary to cover your expenses and loan repayments!

Creative Payment and Repayment

As medical school debt climbs, some private practices and hospitals are using bonuses to attract educationally indentured young M.D.'s.

The "Northern Exposure" Plan

Some medical students are making arrangements with hometown hospitals to pay their medical school tuition. This comes with an agreement that the doctor return there to practice for a specified period of time. Agreements are signed converting tuition payment to a loan if the doctor fails to fulfill the obligation.

Group Practices

Medical groups are also getting wise to the loan repayment woes of new physicians. It is not uncommon now for a large group to offer loan repayment options to lure new doctors who have amassed a large debt. Practicing physicians (who are good risks to lenders) can do this by securing a low-interest private loan at, or just above, the prime rate. They use the loan to pay off the higher interest loan and let the new doctor pay off the lower interest loan. The beauty of this arrangement is that the loan secured by the practice is a business loan and, therefore, tax deductible by the practice.

Just the Facts

The AAMC Data Book is a good place to begin considering your projected earnings vs. your projected debt. Published annually since 1981, the book contains a variety of statistical information, including:

- Mean tuition and fees for first-year med school educational indebtedness
- Career choices and specialty plans of graduating med students
- Median net income of physicians before taxes and after expenses

To order, contact:

AAMC
Publications Department
2450 N Street, N.W.
Washington, DC 20037
(202) 828-0416
Fax: (202) 828-1123

Bringing Home the Bacon

Although the uncertain world of managed care has made income projections difficult, these statistics can give you a sense of an M.D.'s earning power, in relation to the U.S. national median:

- In 1999, the national median annual earnings for men was $32,136; for women, $24,596.
- In 1973, doctors' average salary was four times greater than the national median; in 1994, it was 8.5 times greater.
- The median income for allopathic physicians in 1997 was $164,000 after expenses.
- In 1997, radiologists made $260,000 after expenses, compared to general practice physicians, who averaged $132,000.

Source: *Occupational Outlook Handbook, 2000–01*

Headhunters

Search firms that place doctors in hard-to-fill practices are also finding ways to use loan repayment as a carrot, encouraging independent practices to tailor debt assistance bonuses to be competitive with HMO's and hospitals that are buying up family practitioners. Some offer a lump sum payout of as much as $25,000. Others provide "earn-out agreements" that spread the practice-paid loan repayment over an agreed upon time, while still others offer a combination of an up-front bonus and an earn-out agreement.

State Loan Forgiveness Programs

Many states have initiated programs of loan repayment for doctors who agree to practice in high-need areas. Some get matching grants from the government to assist physicians in public clinics or private, nonprofit practices. Unfortunately, no federal money is available to assist those doctors going into private practices, although some states may use their own money to do this.

When you're projecting your loan repayments, you need to remember that, while the payments will stay relatively stable, your salary will (presumably) increase over the repayment term of the loan. The loan payments will be less onerous as your salary goes up. On the other hand, the longer you are out of school, the more major expenses you're likely to have: a house, car, children, and so on.

Useful Financial Aid Electronic Resources

There is a significant amount of information available on the World Wide Web that will assist you in planning for the financing of your medical education. You should take advantage of the valuable resources listed below. These sites contain a wealth of information that will help you not only to determine how to apply for funds, but also how to repay loans:

- http://www.aamc.org/stuapps
  American Association of Medical Colleges. Includes information about the MEDLOANS program and debt management for borrowers.

- http://www.salliemae.com
  Homepage of the Student Loan Marketing Association.

- http://www.hrsa.dhhs.gov/bhpr/dsa/
  Health Resources and Services Administration Division of Student Assistance provides this site for health professions financial aid programs.

- http://www.usagroup.com
  Guarantee agency Website for information about borrowing loans. Borrowers can access their loan accounts, which are serviced by USA Group.

- http://www.ed.gov
  U.S. Department of Education.

- http://www.finaid.org
  A very good catch-all financial aid information index sponsored by the National Association of Financial Aid Administrators. Contains many useful links.

- http://www.fastweb.com
  A good source for external scholarship assistance.

Hitting the Road

Congratulations! If you've come this far, you've done a lot of work. You probably have a better sense now of what sort of medical school program is best suited for you, what you can do to get in, and how to pay for your education. Now it's time to take the plunge and contact specific med programs to learn their fine points.

Will My Paycheck Cover My Expenses?

Income

1. My annual salary/wages $ _____

2. My spouse/partner's salary/wages   _____

3. Other income (source/amount) (e.g., interest, self-employment,   _____
   etc.; don't include gifts that may not be available each year)

4. Total annual income (sum of lines 1–3)   _____

5. Monthly income (line 4 divided by 12)   _____

Mandatory Expenses

6. Taxes (assume 1/3 of total monthly income)   _____

7. Monthly mandatory deductions from salary (e.g., health   _____
   insurance, required pension contribution)

8. My monthly student loan payment (assume $125 per $10,000 of student loans) _____

9. My spouse/partner's monthly student loan payment   _____

10. My total monthly personal debt payments (credit card and other personal debts; _____
    assume minimum payment of 3 percent of total credit card balance)

11. My spouse/partner's total monthly personal debt payments   _____

12. Total of what I have to pay each month (sum of lines 6–11)   _____

Discretionary Monthly Income

13. Total monthly income (line 5)   _____

14. Total monthly mandatory expenses (line 12)   _____

15. Monthly total available for living expenses (line 14 minus line 13) _____

Living Expenses/Discretionary Expenses

16. Rent/mortgage and maintenance fees   _____

17. Utilities and phone (local and long distance)   _____

18. Groceries and meals away from home (including lunches at work) _____

19. Clothing, laundry, dry cleaning   _____

20. Medical and dental care, prescriptions   _____

21. Recreation, entertainment (also include newspapers, magazines, TV/cable) _____

22. Car (payments, parking, gas, insurance, repairs) or mass transit expenses _____

23. Vacation/travel   _____

24. Dependent or child care   _____

25. Insurance (home, life, medical, dental, renter's)   _____

26. Personal care   _____

27. Gifts, miscellaneous   _____

28. Savings, emergency fund, retirement (emergency fund should equal 3–6 mo. salary; _____
    recommended level of savings/retirement investment = 10% of gross monthly income)

29. Total monthly living and discretionary expenses (sum of lines 16–28) _____

30. Total monthly amount of money remaining and available for savings, investment, _____
    improved life style (line 15 minus line 29)

31. Annual amount of money remaining (line 30 times 12)   _____

Medical Schools

Allopathic Medical Schools

UNITED STATES

Alabama

UNIVERSITY OF ALABAMA

School of Medicine
Medical Student Services
VHP-100
1530 3rd Avenue South
Birmingham, AL 35294-0019
Phone: (205) 934-2330
Fax: (205) 934-8724
E-mail: admissions@uasom.meis.uab.edu
http://main.uab.edu/uasom/
Application: AMCAS
Deadline: November 1
Type of School: Public

UNIVERSITY OF SOUTH ALABAMA

College of Medicine
Office of Admissions
2015 Medical Science Building
Mobile, AL 36688-0002
Phone: (334) 460-7176
http://southmed.usouthal.edu/
Application: AMCAS
Deadline: November 15
Type of School: Public

Arizona

UNIVERSITY OF ARIZONA

College of Medicine
Admissions Office, Box 245075
Tucson, AZ 85724-5075
Phone: (520) 626-6214
http://www.medicine.arizona.edu
Application: AMCAS
Deadline: November 1
Type of School: Public

Arkansas

UNIVERSITY OF ARKANSAS

College of Medicine
Office of Student Admissions
Slot 551, 4301 West Markham Street
Little Rock, AR 72205-7199
Phone: (501) 686-5354
E-mail: SouthTomG@exchange.uams.edu
http://www.uams.edu/com/
Application: AMCAS
Deadline: November 1
Type of School: Public

California

DREW/UCLA JOINT MEDICAL PROGRAM

Drew University of Medicine and Science
1621 East 120 Street
Los Angeles, CA 90059
Phone: (323) 563-4952
E-mail: admsn@cdrewu.edu
http://www.cdrewu.edu/
Application: AMCAS
Deadline: November 15
Type of School: Public

LOMA LINDA UNIVERSITY

School of Medicine
Admissions Office
Loma Linda, CA 92350
Phone: (909) 558-4467
(800) 422-4558
E-mail: ledwards@som.llu.edu
http://www.llu.edu/llu/medicine/
Application: AMCAS
Deadline: November 1
Type of School: Private

STANFORD UNIVERSITY

School of Medicine
Office of Admissions
851 Welch Road, Suite 154
Palo Alto, CA 94304-1677
Phone: (650) 723-6861
Fax: (650) 725-4599
http://med-www.stanford.edu/
Application: AMCAS
Deadline: November 1
Type of School: Private

UNIVERSITY OF CALIFORNIA—DAVIS

School of Medicine
Admissions Office
One Shields Avenue
Davis, CA 95616
Phone: (530) 752-2717
E-mail: medadmsinfo@ucdavis.edu
http://www-med.ucdavis.edu/

Application: AMCAS
Deadline: November 1
Type of School: Public

UNIVERSITY OF CALIFORNIA—IRVINE

College of Medicine
Office of Admissions and Outreach
Medical Education Building 802
Irvine, CA 92697-4089
Phone: (800) 824-5388
(949) 824-5388
E-mail: mmcclell@uci.edu
http://www.com.uci.edu
Application: AMCAS
Deadline: November 1
Type of School: Public

UNIVERSITY OF CALIFORNIA—LOS ANGELES

School of Medicine
Admissions Office
12-109 Center for the Health Sciences
Box 957035
Los Angeles, CA 90095-7035
Phone: (310) 825-6081
E-mail: admissions@deans.medsch.ucla.edu
http://www.medsch.ucla.edu/
Application: AMCAS
Deadline: November 1
Type of School: Public

UNIVERSITY OF CALIFORNIA—SAN DIEGO

School of Medicine
Office of Admissions, Dept. 0621
9500 Gilman Drive
La Jolla, CA 92093-0621
Phone: (858) 534-3880
Fax: (858) 534-5282
E-mail: somadmissions@ucsd.edu
http://www.medicine.ucsd.edu/
Application: AMCAS
Deadline: November 1
Type of School: Public

UNIVERSITY OF CALIFORNIA—
SAN FRANCISCO

School of Medicine
Office of Admission, C-200
Box 0408
San Francisco, CA 94143-0408
Phone: (415) 476-4044
http://www.som.ucsf.edu
Application: AMCAS
Deadline: November 1
Type of School: Public

UNIVERSITY OF SOUTHERN CALIFORNIA

Keck School of Medicine
Office of Admissions
1975 Zonal Avenue, KAM 100-C
Los Angeles, CA 90089
Phone: (323) 442-2552
Fax: (323) 442-2433
E-mail: medadmit@hsc.usc.edu
http://www.usc.edu/medicine/
Application: AMCAS
Deadline: November 1
Type of School: Private

Colorado

UNIVERSITY OF COLORADO

School of Medicine
Medical School Admissions
4200 East 9th Avenue, C-297
Denver, CO 80262
Phone: (303) 315-7361
Fax: (303) 315-8494
http://www.uchsc.edu/sm/sm/
Application: AMCAS
Deadline: November 1
Type of School: Public

Connecticut

UNIVERSITY OF CONNECTICUT

School of Medicine
Room AG031
Mail Code: MC 3906
263 Farmington Avenue
Farmington, CT 06030
Phone: (860) 679-4306
Fax: (860) 679-7699
E-mail: barta@adp.uchc.edu
http://www.uchc.edu/
Application: AMCAS
Deadline: December 15
Type of School: Public

YALE UNIVERSITY

School of Medicine
Office of Admissions
367 Cedar Street
New Haven, CT 06510
Phone: (203) 785-2696
Fax: (203) 785-3234
E-mail: medical.admissions@yale.edu
http://info.med.yale.edu/medadmit
Deadline: October 15
Type of School: Private

District of Columbia

GEORGE WASHINGTON UNIVERSITY

School of Medicine and Health Sciences
Office of Admissions
2300 I Street, NW, Room 615
Washington, DC 20037
Phone: (202) 994-3506
Fax: (202) 994-1753
E-mail: medadmit@gwis2.circ.gwu.edu
http://www.gwumc.edu/smhs
Application: AMCAS
Deadline: December 1
Type of School: Private

GEORGETOWN UNIVERSITY

School of Medicine
Office of Admissions
3900 Reservoir Road, NW
Washington, DC 20007-2195
Phone: (202) 687-1154
Fax: (202) 687-7143
http://www.dml.georgetown.edu/schmed/
Application: AMCAS
Deadline: November 1
Type of School: Private

HOWARD UNIVERSITY

College of Medicine
Admissions Office
520 W Street, NW
Washington, DC 20059
Phone: (202) 806-6270
Fax: (202) 806-7934
http://www.med.howard.edu
Application: AMCAS
Deadline: December 15
Type of School: Private

Florida

FLORIDA STATE UNIVERSITY

Program in Medical Sciences
104 SCN
Tallahassee, FL 32306-4300
Phone: (850) 644-1855
Fax: (850) 644-5766
E-mail: pims@mailer.fsu.edu
http://www.fsu.edu/~pims/pims.html
Application: AMCAS
Deadline: December 15
Type of School: Public

UNIVERSITY OF FLORIDA

College of Medicine
Chair, Medical Selection Committee
J. Hillis Miller Health Center
Gainesville, FL 32610
Phone: (352) 392-4569
Fax: (352) 392-1307

E-mail: robyn@dean.med.ufl.edu
http://www.med.ufl.edu/
Application: AMCAS
Deadline: December 1
Type of School: Public

UNIVERSITY OF MIAMI

School of Medicine
Office of Admissions
P.O. Box 016159
Miami, FL 33101
Phone: (305) 243-6791
E-mail: med.admissions@miami.edu
http://www.med.miami.edu/
Application: AMCAS
Deadline: December 15
Type of School: Private

UNIVERSITY OF SOUTH FLORIDA

College of Medicine
Office of Admissions, Box 3
12901 Bruce B. Downs Blvd.
Tampa, FL 33612-4799
Phone: (813) 974-2229
Fax: (813) 974-4990
http://www.med.usf.edu/med.html
Application: AMCAS
Deadline: December 1
Type of School: Public

Georgia

EMORY UNIVERSITY

School of Medicine
Woodruff Health Sciences Center
Administration Building,
Admissions, Room 303
Atlanta, GA 30322-4510
Phone: (404) 727-5660
Fax: (404) 727-5456
E-mail: medschadmiss@medadm.emory.edu
http://www.emory.edu/WHSC/MED/med.html
Application: AMCAS
Deadline: October 15
Type of School: Private

MEDICAL COLLEGE OF GEORGIA

School of Medicine
Associate Dean for Admissions
Room AA2040
Augusta, GA 30912-4760
Phone: (706) 721-3186
Fax: (706) 721-0959
E-mail: stdadmin.stdadmin@mail.mcg.edu
http://www.mcg.edu/som/index.html
Application: AMCAS
Deadline: November 1
Type of School: Public

MERCER UNIVERSITY

School of Medicine
Office of Admissions and Student Affairs
1550 College Street
Macon, GA 31207
Phone: (912) 301-2542
Fax: (912) 301-2547
E-mail: admissions@gain.mercer.edu
http://168.17.205.219/musm/default.asp
Application: AMCAS
Deadline: November 1
Type of School: Private

MOREHOUSE SCHOOL OF MEDICINE

Admissions and Student Affairs
720 Westview Drive, SW
Atlanta, GA 30310
Phone: (404) 752-1650
Fax: (404) 752-1512
E-mail: catalog@msm.edu
http://www.msm.edu
Aplication: AMCAS
Deadline: December 1
Type of School: Private

Hawaii

UNIVERSITY OF HAWAII

John A. Burns School of Medicine
Office of Admissions
1960 East - West Road, B104
Honolulu, HI 96822
Phone: (808) 956-8300
Fax: (808) 956-9547
E-mail: nishikim@jabsom.biomed.hawaii.edu
http://medworld.biomed.hawaii.edu/
Application: AMCAS
Deadline: December 1
Type of Application: Public

Illinois

FINCH UNIVERSITY OF HEALTH SCIENCES

Chicago Medical School
Office of Admissions
3333 Green Bay Road
North Chicago, IL 60064-3095
Phone: (847) 578-3205
Fax: (847) 578-3284
http://www.finchcms.edu/cms/medschool.html
Application: AMCAS
Deadline: November 15
Type of School: Private

LOYOLA UNIVERSITY OF CHICAGO

Stritch School of Medicine
Office of Admissions
2160 South First Avenue
Maywood, IL 60153
Phone: (708) 216-3229
http://www.meddean.luc.edu/
Application: AMCAS
Deadline: November 15
Type of School: Private

NORTHWESTERN UNIVERSITY

Medical School
Admissions Office
Morton Building 1-606
303 East Chicago Avenue
Chicago, IL 60611-3008
Phone: (312) 503-8206
E-mail: med-admissions@nwu.edu
http://www.nums.nwu.edu/
Application: AMCAS
Deadline: October 15
Type of School: Private

RUSH MEDICAL COLLEGE

Office of Admissions
Suite 524
600 South Paulina Street
Chicago, IL 60612
Phone: (312) 942-6913
Fax: (312) 942-2333
E-mail: medcol@rush.edu
http://www.rushu.rush.edu/medcol
Application: AMCAS
Deadline: November 15
Type of School: Private

SOUTHERN ILLINOIS UNIVERSITY

School of Medicine
Office of Student and Alumni Affairs
P.O. Box 19624
Springfield, IL 62794-9624
Phone: (217) 524-6013
http://www.siumed.edu/admiss.htlm
Application: AMCAS
Deadline: November 15
Type of School: Public

UNIVERSITY OF CHICAGO

Pritzker School of Medicine
Office of the Dean of Students
924 East 57th Street, Suite 104
Chicago, IL 60637-5416
Phone: (773) 702-1939
Fax: (773) 702-2598
http://pritzer.bsd.uchicago.edu
Application: AMCAS
Deadline: November 15
Type of School: Private

UNIVERSITY OF ILLINOIS

College of Medicine
Office of Medical College Admissions
1853 West Polk MC/785
Chicago, IL 60612
Phone: (312) 996-5635
Fax: (312) 996-6693
http://www.uic.edu/depts/mcam/
Application: AMCAS
Deadline: December 15
Type of School: Public

Indiana

INDIANA UNIVERSITY

School of Medicine
Medical School Admissions Office
Fesler Hall 213
1120 South Drive
Indianapolis, IN 46202-5113
Phone: (317) 274-3772
Fax: (317) 278-0211
E-mail: inmedadm@iupui.edu
http://www.medicine.iu.edu/home.html
Application: AMCAS
Deadline: December 15
Type of School: Public

Iowa

UNIVERSITY OF IOWA

College of Medicine
Office of Student Affairs
100 Medicine Administration Building
Iowa City, IA 52242-1101
Phone: (319) 335-8052
(800)553-IOWA
Fax: (319) 335-8049
E-mail: medical-admissions@uiowa.edu
http://www.medicine.uiowa.edu/
Application: AMCAS
Deadline: November 1
Type of School: Public

Kansas

UNIVERSITY OF KANSAS

Medical Center
School of Medicine
Admissions Department
3901 Rainbow Blvd.
Kansas City, KS 66160
Phone: (913) 588-5245
Fax: (913) 588-5259
E-mail: mheinen@kumc.edu
http://www.kumc.edu/som/som.html
Application: AMCAS
Deadline: October 15
Type of School: Public

Kentucky

UNIVERSITY OF KENTUCKY

College of Medicine
Chandler Medical Center
800 Rose Street
Admissions, Room MN-102
Lexington, KY 40536-0298
Phone: (606) 323-6161
Fax: (606) 323-2076
http://www.comed.uky.edu/medicine
Application: AMCAS
Deadline: November 1
Type of School: Public

UNIVERSITY OF LOUISVILLE

School of Medicine
Office of Admissions
Abell Administration Center
323 E. Chestnut Street
Louisville, KY 40202-3866
Phone: (502) 852-5193
E-mail: medadm@louisville.edu
http://www.louisville.edu/medschool
Application: AMCAS
Deadline: November 1
Type of School: Public

Louisiana

LOUISIANA STATE UNIVERSITY—NEW ORLEANS

School of Medicine in New Orleans
Admissions Office
1901 Perdido Street, Box P3-4
New Orleans, LA 70112-1393
Phone: (504) 568-6262
E-mail: ms-admissions@lsumc.edu/
http://www.medschool.lsumc.edu/admissions
Application: AMCAS
Deadline: November 15
Type of School: Public

LOUISIANA STATE UNIVERSITY—SHREVEPORT

School of Medicine
Office of Student Admissions
P.O. Box 33932
Shreveport, LA 71130-3932
Phone: (318) 675-5190
Fax: (318) 675-5244
E-mail: shvadm@lsumc.edu
http://www.sh.lsumc.edu/
Application: AMCAS
Deadline: November 15
Type of School: Public

TULANE UNIVERSITY

School of Medicine
Office of Admissions
1430 Tulane Ave, SL67
New Orleans, LA 70112-2699
Phone: (504) 588-5187
Fax: (504) 988-6735
E-mail: medsch@tmcpop.tmc.tulane.edu
http://www.tmc.tulane.edu
Application: AMCAS
Deadline: December 15
Type of School: Private

Maryland

JOHNS HOPKINS UNIVERSITY

School of Medicine
Committee on Admission
720 Rutland Avenue, Room 109
Baltimore, MD 21205-2196
Phone: (410) 955-3182
http://www.med.jhu.edu/admissions/
Application: AMCAS
Deadline: October 15
Type of School: Private

UNIVERSITY OF MARYLAND

School of Medicine
Committee on Admissions Room 1-005
655 West Baltimore Street
Baltimore, MD 21201
Phone: (410) 706-7478
http://www.som1.umaryland.edu/
Application: AMCAS
Deadline: November 1
Type of School: Public

UNIFORMED SERVICES UNIVERSITY OF THE HEALTH SCIENCES

F. Edward Hébert School of Medicine
Admissions Office
Room A-1041
4301 Jones Bridge Road
Bethesda, MD 20814-4799
Phone: (301) 295-310
(800) 772-1743
Fax: (301) 295-3545
E-mail: admissions@mxa.usuhs.mil
http://www.usuhs.mil/admis/admissions.html
Application: AMCAS
Deadline: November 1
Type of School: Federally chartered

Massachussetts

BOSTON UNIVERSITY

School of Medicine
Admissions Office
715 Albany Street, L-124
Boston, MA 02118
Phone: (617) 638-4630
http://www.bumc.bu.edu/
Application: AMCAS
Deadline: November 15
Type of School: Private

HARVARD MEDICAL SCHOOL

Office of Admissions
25 Shattuck Street
Boston, MA 02115-6092
Phone: (617) 432-1550
E-mail: admissions_office@hms.harvard.edu
http://www.hms.harvard.edu/
Application: AMCAS
Deadline: October 15
Type of School: Private

TUFTS UNIVERSITY

School of Medicine
Office of Admissions
136 Harrison Avenue
Boston, MA 02111
Phone: (617) 636-6571
http://www.tufts.edu/med/
Application: AMCAS
Deadline: November 1
Type of School: Private

UNIVERSITY OF MASSACHUSETTS MEDICAL SCHOOL

Associate Dean for Admissions
55 Lake Avenue, North
Worcester, MA 01655
Phone: (508) 856-2323
Fax: (508) 856-3629
http://www.umassmed.edu/
Application: AMCAS
Deadline: November 1
Type of School: Public

Michigan

MICHIGAN STATE UNIVERSITY

College of Human Medicine
Office of Admissions
A-239 Life Sciences
East Lansing, MI 48824-1317
Phone: (517) 353-9620
Fax: (517) 432-0021
E-mail: MDAdmissions@msu.edu
http://www.chm.msu.edu/
Application: AMCAS
Deadline: November 15
Type of Schol: Public

UNIVERSITY OF MICHIGAN MEDICAL SCHOOL

Admissions Office
M4130 Medical Sciences, Building I
1301 Catherine
Ann Arbor, MI 48109-0611
Phone: (734) 764-6317
http://www.med.umich.edu/medschool/bulletin/admission.html
Application: AMCAS
Deadline: November 15
Type of Schol: Public

WAYNE STATE UNIVERSITY

School of Medicine
Director of Admissions
1310 Scott Hall
540 East Canfield
Detroit, MI 48201
Phone: (313) 577-1466
Fax: (313) 577-1330
E-mail: dstreet@med.wayne.edu
http://www.med.wayne.edu/
Application: AMCAS
Deadline: December 15
Type of School: Public

Minnesota

MAYO MEDICAL SCHOOL

Admissions Committee
200 First Street, SW
Rochester, MN 55905
Phone: (507) 284-3671
Fax: (507) 284-2634
E-mail: morris.leibert@mayo.edu
http://www.mayo.edu/education/mms/
Application: AMCAS
Deadline: November 1
Type of School: Private

UNIVERSITY OF MINNESOTA—DULUTH

School of Medicine
Office of Admissions, Room 107
10 University Drive
Duluth, MN 55812
Phone: (218) 726-8511
Fax: (218) 726-6235
E-mail: jcarls10@d.umn.edu
http://www.d.umn.edu/medweb/admissions
Application: AMCAS
Deadline: November 15
Type of School: Public

UNIVERSITY OF MINNESOTA

Medical School
Office of Admissions and Student Affairs
Box 293 - UMHC
420 Delaware Street, SE
Minneapolis, MN 55455-0310
Phone: (612) 624-1188
Fax: (612) 626-4200
http://www.med.umn.edu/
Application: AMCAS
Deadline: November 15
Type of School: Public

Mississippi

UNIVERSITY OF MISSISSIPPI

School of Medicine
Chair, Admissions Committee
2500 North State Street
Jackson, MS 39216-4505
Phone: (601) 984-5010
Fax: (601) 984-5008
http://umc.edu/medicine
Application: AMCAS
Deadline: November 1
Type of Application: Public

Missouri

ST. LOUIS UNIVERSITY

School of Medicine
Admissions Committee
1402 South Grand Blvd.
St. Louis, MO 63104
Phone: (314) 577-8205
Fax: (314) 577-8214
E-mail: medadmis@slu.edu
http://www.slu.edu/colleges/med/
Application: AMCAS
Deadline: December 15
Type of School: Private

UNIVERSITY OF MISSOURI—COLUMBIA

School of Medicine
Office of Admissions
MA202 Medical Sciences Bldg.
One Hospital Drive
Columbia, MO 65212
Phone: (573) 882-2923
Fax: (573) 884-4808
E-mail: nolkej@health.missouri.edu
http://www.hsc.missouri.edu/~medicine/
Application: AMCAS
Deadline: November 1
Type of School: Public

UNIVERSITY OF MISSOURI—KANSAS CITY

School of Medicine
Council on Selection
2411 Holmes
Kansas City, MO 64108
Phone: (816) 235-1870
Fax: (816) 235-5277
http://research.med.umkc.edu/
Deadline: November 15
Type of School: Public

WASHINGTON UNIVERSITY

School of Medicine
Office of Admissions
660 S. Euclid Ave., Campus Box 8107
St. Louis, MO 63110
Phone: (314) 362-6858
Fax: (314) 362-4658
E-mail: wumscoa@msnotes.wust1.edu
http://medschool.wustl.edu/admissions/
Application: AMCAS
Deadline: December 1
Type of School: Private

Nebraska

CREIGHTON UNIVERSITY

School of Medicine
Office of Admissions
2500 California Plaza
Omaha, NE 68178
Phone: (402) 280-2798
Fax: (402) 280-1241
E-mail: medschadm@creighton.edu
http://medicine.creighton.edu/
Application: AMCAS
Deadline: December 1
Type of School: Private

UNIVERSITY OF NEBRASKA

College of Medicine
Office of Academic and Student Affairs
986585 Nebraska Medical Center
Omaha, NE 68198-6585
Phone: (402) 559-2259

Fax: (402) 559-4148
E-mail: jmeyers@unmc.edu
http://www.unmc.edu/
Application: AMCAS
Deadline: November 1
Type of School: Public

Nevada

UNIVERSITY OF NEVADA

School of Medicine
Office of Admissions and Student Affairs Mail Stop 357
Reno, NV 89557
Phone: (775) 784-6063
Fax: (775) 784-6194
http://www.unr.edu/med/
Application: AMCAS
Deadline: November 1
Type of School: Public

New Hampshire

DARTMOUTH MEDICAL SCHOOL

Office of Admissions
7020 Remsen, Room 306
Hanover, NH 03755-3833
Phone: (603) 650-1505
E-mail: DMS.Admissions@Dartmouth.edu
http://www.dartmouth.edu/dms/
Application: AMCAS
Deadline: November 1
Type of School: Private

New Jersey

UMDNJ—NEW JERSEY MEDICAL SCHOOL

Office of Admissions
185 South Orange Avenue, C653
Newark, NJ 07103-2714
Phone: (973) 972-4631
Fax: (973) 972-7986
E-mail: njmsadmiss@umdnj.edu
http://www.umdnj.edu/njmsweb/
Application: AMCAS
Deadline: December 1
Type of School: Public

UMDNJ—R. W. JOHNSON MEDICAL SCHOOL

Office of Admissions
675 Hoes Lane
Piscataway, NJ 08854-5635
Phone: (732) 235-4576
Fax: (732) 235-5078
http://www2.umdnj.edu/rwjpweb
Application: AMCAS
Deadline: December 1
Type of School: Public

New Mexico

UNIVERSITY OF NEW MEXICO

School of Medicine
Office of Admissions and Student Affairs
Basic Medical Sciences Building
Room 107
Albuquerque, NM 87131-5166
Phone: (505) 272-4766
Fax: (505) 272-8239
http://hsc.unm.edu/som/
Application: AMCAS
Deadline: November 15
Type of School: Public

New York

ALBANY MEDICAL COLLEGE

Office of Admissions
Mail Code 3
47 New Scotland Avenue
Albany, NY 12208-3479
Phone: (518) 262-5521
Fax: (518) 262-5887
http://www.amc.edu/academic/college/college.html
Application: AMCAS
Deadline: November 15
Type of School: Private

ALBERT EINSTEIN COLLEGE OF MEDICINE

Office of Admissions
Jack and Pearl Resnick Campus
1300 Morris Park Avenue

Bronx, NY 10461
Phone: (718) 430-2106
E-mail: admissions@aecom.yu.edu
http://www.aecom.yu.edu/
Application: AMCAS
Deadline: November 1
Type of School: Private

COLUMBIA UNIVERSITY

College of Physicians and Surgeons
Admissions Office, Room 1-416
630 West 168th Street
New York, NY 10032
Phone: (212) 305-3595
Fax: (212) 305-3601
E-mail: pt8@columbia.edu
http://cpmcnet.columbia.edu/dept/ps/
Deadline: October 15
Type of School: Private

CORNELL UNIVERSITY MEDICAL COLLEGE

Office of Admissions
Weill Medical College of Cornell University
445 East 69th Street
New York, NY 10021
Phone: (212) 746-1067
Fax: (212) 746-8052
E-mail: cumc-admissions@mail.med.cornell.edu
http://www.med.cornell.edu/
Application: AMCAS
Deadline: October 15
Type of School: Private

MOUNT SINAI SCHOOL OF MEDICINE

Director of Admissions
Annenberg Bldg. Room 5-04
One Gustave L. Levy Place, Box 1002
New York, NY 10029-6574
Phone: (212) 241-6696
Fax: (212) 828-4135
E-mail: admissions@mssm.edu
http://www.mssm.edu/
Application: AMCAS
Deadline: November 1
Type of School: Private

NEW YORK MEDICAL COLLEGE

Office of Admissions
Room 127, Sunshine Cottage
Valhalla, NY 10595
Phone: (914) 594-4507
Fax: (914) 594-4976
http://www.nymc.edu/
Application: AMCAS
Deadline: December 1
Type of School: Private

NEW YORK UNIVERSITY

School of Medicine
Office of Admissions
P.O. Box 1924
New York, NY 10016
Phone: (212) 263-5290
http://www.med.nyu.edu/
Deadline: November 17
Type of School: Private

STATE UNIVERSITY OF NEW YORK— BROOKLYN

SUNY Downstate College of Medicine
Director of Admissions
450 Clarkson Avenue, Box 60M
Brooklyn, NY 11203
Phone: (718) 270-2446
E-mail: admissions@netmail.hscbklyn.edu
http://md.hscbklyn.edu/
Application: AMCAS
Deadline: December 15
Type of School: Public

STATE UNIVERSITY OF NEW YORK— UNIVERSITY AT BUFFALO

School of Medicine and Biomedical Sciences
Office of Medical Admissions
45 Biomedical Education Building
Buffalo, NY 14214-3013
Phone: (716) 829-3466
Fax: (716) 829-3849
E-mail: jjrosso@acsu.buffalo.edu
http://www.smbs.buffalo.edu/ome/admissio.htm
Application: AMCAS
Deadlne: November 1
Type of School: Public

STATE UNIVERSITY OF NEW YORK— STONY BROOK

School of Medicine
Office of Admissions
Health Sciences Center, 4L
Stony Brook, NY 11794-8434
Phone: (516) 444-2113
E-mail: admissions@dean.som.sunysb.edu
http://www.hsc.sunysb.edu/som/
Application: AMCAS
Deadline: November 15
Type of School: Public

STATE UNIVERSITY OF NEW YORK— SYRACUSE

SUNY Upstate College of Medicine
Office of Student Admissions
SUNY Health Sciences Center
750 East Adams St., CAB Rm. 204
Syracuse, NY 13210-2339
Phone: (315) 464-4570
Fax: (315) 464-8867
E-mail: admiss@hscsyr.edu
http://www.hscsyr.edu/
Application: AMCAS
Deadline: November 1
Type of School: Public

UNIVERSITY OF ROCHESTER

School of Medicine and Dentistry
Director of Admissions
Medical Center Box 601-A
Rochester, NY 14642
Phone: (716) 275-4539
Fax: (716) 273-1016
E-mail: mdadmish@urmc.rochester.edu
http://www.urmc.rochester.edu/smd/
Application: AMCAS
Deadline: October 15
Type of School: Private

North Carolina

DUKE UNIVERSITY

School of Medicine
Committee on Admissions
P.O. Box 3710
Durham, NC 27710
Phone: (919) 684-2985
Fax: (919) 684-8893
http://www2.mc.duke.edu/depts/som
Application: AMCAS
Deadline: November 1
Type of School: Private

EAST CAROLINA UNIVERSITY

Office of Admissions
School of Medicine
Greenville, NC 27858-4354
Phone: (252) 816-2202
http://www.med.ecu.edu/
Application: AMCAS
Deadline: November 15
Type of School: Public

UNIVERSITY OF NORTH CAROLINA— CHAPEL HILL

School of Medicine
Admissions Office
CB# 7000 121 MacNider Bldg.
Chapel Hill, NC 27599-7000
Phone: (919) 962-8331
Fax: (919) 966-9930
E-mail: esmann@med.unc.edu
http://www.med.unc.edu
Application: AMCAS
Deadline: November 15
Type of School: Public

WAKE FOREST UNIVERSITY SCHOOL OF MEDICINE

Office of Medical School Admissions
Medical Center Blvd.
Winston-Salem, NC 27157-1090
Phone: (336) 716-4264

Fax: (336) 716-5807
E-mail: medadmit@wfubmc.edu
http://www.wfubmc.edu/
Application: AMCAS
Deadline: November 1
Type of School: Private

North Dakota

UNIVERSITY OF NORTH DAKOTA

School of Medicine and Health Sciences
Secretary, Committee on Admissions
501 North Columbia Road, Box 9037
Grand Forks, ND 58202-9037
Phone: (701) 777-4221
Fax: (701) 777-4942
E-mail: jdemers@medicine.nodak.edu
http://www.med.und.nodak.edu/
Deadline: November 1
Type of School: Public

Ohio

CASE WESTERN RESERVE UNIVERSITY

School of Medicine
Admissions and Student Affairs
10900 Euclid Avenue
Cleveland, OH 44106-4920
Phone: (216) 368-3450
Fax: (216) 368-6011
E-mail: ack@po.cwru.edu
http://medisvww.meds.cwru.edu/
Application: AMCAS
Deadline: November 1
Type of School: Private

MEDICAL COLLEGE OF OHIO

Admissions Office
3045 Arlington Avenue
Toledo, OH 43614
Phone: (419) 383-4229
Fax: (419) 383-4005
http://www.mco.edu/
Application: AMCAS
Deadline: November 1
Type of School: Public

NORTHEASTERN OHIO UNIVERSITIES

College of Medicine
Office of Admissions and Educational Research
P.O. Box 95
Rootstown, OH 44272-0095
Phone: (330) 325-6270
Fax: (330) 325-8372
E-mail: admission@neoucom.edu
http://www.neoucom.edu/
Application: AMCAS
Deadline: November 1
Type of School: Public

OHIO STATE UNIVERSITY

The Ohio State University College of Medicine & Public Health
Admissions Committee
270-A Meiling Hall
370 West Ninth Avenue
Columbus, OH 43210-1238
Phone: (614) 292-7137
Fax: (614) 292-1544
E-mail: admiss-med@osu.edu
http://www.med.ohio-state.edu/
Application: AMCAS
Deadline: November 1
Type of School: Public

UNIVERSITY OF CINCINNATI

College of Medicine
Office of Student Affairs/Admissions
P.O. Box 670552
Cincinnati, OH 45267-0552
Phone: (513) 558-7314
Fax: (513) 558-1165
http://www.med.uc.edu/
Application: AMCAS
Deadline: November 15
Type of School: Public

WRIGHT STATE UNIVERSITY

School of Medicine
Office of Student Affairs/Admissions
P.O. Box 1751
Dayton, OH 45401
Phone: (937) 775-2934
Fax: (937) 775-3322

E-mail: som_saa@wright.edu
http://www.med.wright.edu/
Application: AMCAS
Deadline: November 15
Type of School: Public

Oklahoma

UNIVERSITY OF OKLAHOMA COLLEGE OF MEDICINE

P.O. Box 26901
Oklahoma City, OK 73190
Phone: (405) 271-2331
Fax: (405) 271-3032
E-mail: admissions@ouhsc.edu
http://www.medicine.ouhsc.edu/
Application: AMCAS
Deadline: October 15
Type of School: Public

Oregon

OREGON HEALTH SCIENCES UNIVERSITY

School of Medicine
Office of the Dean
3181 SW Sam Jackson Park Road, L102
Portland, OR 97201
Phone: (503) 494-2998
Fax: (503) 494-3400
http://www.ohsu.edu/som/
Application: AMCAS
Deadline: October 15
Type of School: Public

Pennsylvania

ALLEGHENY UNIVERSITY OF THE HEALTH SCIENCES

(formerly Medical College of Pennsylvania and Hahnemann University)
MCP Hahnemann School of Medicine
Admissions Office
2900 Queen Lane
Philadelphia, PA 19129

E-mail: MCPHU.MedAdmissions@drexel.edu
Phone: (215) 991-8202
Fax: (215) 843-1766
http://www.auhs.edu/medschool/medschl.html
Application: AMCAS
Deadline: December 1
Type of School: Private

JEFFERSON MEDICAL COLLEGE

Associate Dean for Admissions
1015 Walnut Street, 110 Curtis Bldg.
Philadelphia, PA 19107
Phone: (215) 955-6983
Fax: (215) 955-5151
E-mail: JMC.admissions@mail.tju.edu
http://jeffline.tju.edu/CWIS/JMC
Application: AMCAS
Deadline: November 15
Type of School: Private

PENNSYLVANIA STATE UNIVERSITY

College of Medicine
Office of Student Affairs
P.O. Box 850
Hershey, PA 17033
Phone: (717) 531-8755
Fax: (717) 531-6225
E-mail: hmcstaff@psu.edu
http://www.collmed.psu.edu/
Application: AMCAS
Deadline: November 15
Type of School: Private

TEMPLE UNIVERSITY

School of Medicine
Admissions Office
Suite 305, Student Faculty Center
3340 N. Broad Street
Philadelphia, PA 19140
Phone: (215) 707-3656
Fax: (215) 707-6932
E-mail: gmorton@nimbus.ocis.temple.edu
http://www.temple.edu/medschool/
Application: AMCAS
Deadline: December 1
Type of School: Private

UNIVERSITY OF PENNSYLVANIA

School of Medicine
Director of Admissions and Financial Aid
Stemmler Hall, Suite 100
Philadelphia, PA 19104-6056
Phone: (215) 898-8001
Fax: (215) 573-6645
E-mail: admiss@med.upenn.edu
http://www.med.upenn.edu/
Application: AMCAS
Deadline: November 1
Type of School: Private

UNIVERSITY OF PITTSBURGH

School of Medicine
Office of Admissions
518 Scaife Hall
Pittsburgh, PA 15261
Phone: (412) 648-9891
Fax: (412) 648-8768
E-mail: admissions@fs1.dean-med.pitt.edu
http://www.dean-med.pitt.edu/
Application: AMCAS
Deadline: December 1
Type of School: Private

Puerto Rico

PONCE SCHOOL OF MEDICINE

Admissions Office, P.O. Box 7004
Ponce, PR 00732
Phone: (787) 840-2511
Application: AMCAS
Deadline: December 15
Type of School: Private

UNIVERSIDAD CENTRAL DEL CARIBE

School of Medicine
Office of Admissions
Ramon Ruiz Arnau University Hospital
Call Box 60-327
Bayamón, PR 00960-6032
Phone: (787) 740-1611 ext 210
http://www.uccaribe.edu/
Application: AMCAS
Deadline: December 15
Type of School: Private

UNIVERSITY OF PUERTO RICO

School of Medicine
Central Admissions Office
Medical Sciences Campus
P.O. Box 365067
San Juan, PR 00936-5067
Phone: (787) 758-2525, ext. 5213
E-mail: r_aponte@rcmaxp.upr.clu.edu
http://wwwrcm.upr.clu.edu/
Application: AMCAS
Deadline: December 1
Type of School: Public

Rhode Island

BROWN UNIVERSITY

School of Medicine
Office of Admissions and Financial Aid
97 Waterman St., Box G-A212
Providence, RI 02912-9706
Phone: (401) 863-2149
Fax: (401) 863-3801
E-mail: MedSchool_Admissions@brown.edu
http://biomed.brown.edu
Deadline: March 1
Type of School: Private

South Carolina

MEDICAL UNIVERSITY OF SOUTH CAROLINA

Office of Enrollment Services
171 Ashley Avenue
Charleston, SC 29425
Phone: (843) 792-2055
E-mail: taylorwl@musc.edu
http://www2.musc.edu/medicine.html
Application: AMCAS
Deadline: December 1
Type of School: Public

UNIVERSITY OF SOUTH CAROLINA

School of Medicine
Associate Dean for Medical Education and Academic Affairs
Columbia, SC 29208
Phone: (803) 733-3325

Fax: (803) 733-3328
http://www.med.sc.edu/
Application: AMCAS
Deadline: December 1
Type of School: Public

South Dakota

UNIVERSITY OF SOUTH DAKOTA

School of Medicine
Medical School Admissions
414 Clark St., Room 105
Vermillion, SD 57069
Phone: (605) 677-5233
Fax: (605) 677-5109
http://med.usd.edu/md/
Application: AMCAS
Deadline: November 15
Type of School: Public

Tennessee

EAST TENNESSEE STATE UNIVERSITY

James H. Quillen College of Medicine
Assistant Dean for Admissions and Records
P.O. Box 70580
Johnson City, TN 37614-0580
Phone: (423) 439-4753
Fax: (423) 439-8206
E-mail: sacom@etsu.edu
http://qcom.etsu.edu/
Application: AMCAS
Deadline: December 1
Type of Shcool: Public

MEHARRY MEDICAL COLLEGE

Medical Admissions
Director, Admissions and Records
1005 Dr. D. B. Todd Jr. Boulevard
Nashville, TN 37208-3599
Phone: (615) 327-6223
Fax: (615) 327-6228
E-mail: admissions@mmc.edu
http://www.mmc.edu/
Application: AMCAS
Deadline: December 15
Type of School: Private

UNIVERSITY OF TENNESSEE

College of Medicine
790 Madison Avenue, Room 307
Memphis, TN 38163-2166
Phone: (901) 448-5559
Fax: (901) 448-7255
http://www.utmem.edu/medicine
Application: AMCAS
Deadline: November 15
Type of School: Public

VANDERBILT UNIVERSITY

School of Medicine
Office of Admissions
209 Light Hall
Nashville, TN 37232-0685
Phone: (615) 322-2145
Fax: (615) 343-8397
E-mail: medsch.admis@mcmail.vanderbilt.edu
http://www.mc.Vanderbilt.Edu/medschool
Application: AMCAS
Deadline: October 15
Type of School: Private

Texas

BAYLOR COLLEGE OF MEDICINE

Office of Admissions
One Baylor Plaza
Houston, TX 77030
Phone: (713) 798-4842
Fax: (713) 798-5563
E-mail: melodym@bcm.tmc.edu
http://www.bcm.tmc.edu/
Deadline: November 1
Type of School: Private

TEXAS A&M UNIVERSITY SYSTEM

College of Medicine
Associate Dean for Student Affairs and Admissions
Health Science Center, Room 159
Reynolds Medical Building
College Station, TX 77843-1114
Phone: (409) 845-7743
Fax: (409) 845-5533
E-mail: med-stu-aff@tamu.edu

http://tamushsc.tamu.edu
Application: AMCAS
Deadline: October 1
Type of School: Public

TEXAS TECH UNIVERSITY

School of Medicine
Health Sciences Center
Office of Admissions
Lubbock, TX 79430
Phone: (806) 743-2297
Fax: (806) 743-2725
E-mail: somadm@ttuhsc.edu
http://www.ttuhsc.edu/pages/med.htm
Deadline: October 15
Type of School: Public

UNIVERSITY OF TEXAS—GALVESTON

Medical Branch at Galveston
Office of Admissions
301 University Blvd.
Galveston, TX 77555-1317
Phone: (409) 772-3517
Fax: (409) 747-2909
E-mail:pwylie@utmb.edu/
http://www.utmb.edu/
Application: UTSMDAC
Deadline: October 15
Type of School: Public

UNIVERSITY OF TEXAS—HOUSTON

Medical School at Houston
Office of Admissions, Room G-024
P.O. Box 20708
Houston, TX 77225
Phone: (713) 500-5116
Fax: (713) 500-0604
http://www.med.uth.tmc.edu/
Application: UTSMDAC
Deadline: October 1
Type of School: Public

UNIVERSITY OF TEXAS—SAN ANTONIO

Medical School at San Antonio
Medical School Admissions/Registrar's Office
7703 Floyd Curl Drive
San Antonio, TX 78284-7701
Phone: (210) 567-2665
Fax: (210) 567-2685
http://www.uthscsa.edu/som/som_main.htm
Application: UTSMDAC
Deadline: October 1
Type of School: Public

UNIVERSITY OF TEXAS—SOUTHWESTERN

Southwestern Medical School
Office of the Registrar
5323 Harry Hines Blvd.
Dallas, TX 75235
Phone: (214) 648-5617
Fax: (214) 648-3289
http://www.swmed.edu/
Application: UTSMDAC
Deadline: October 15
Type of School: Public

UNIVERSITY OF TEXAS SYSTEM MEDICAL AND DENTAL APPLICATION CENTER

702 Colorado, Suite 6.400
Austin, TX 78701
Phone (512) 499-4785
Fax (512) 499-4786
E-mail: TMDSAS@utsystem.edu
http://www.utsystem.edu/mdac/

Utah

UNIVERSITY OF UTAH

School of Medicine
Admissions Office
50 North Medical Drive
Salt Lake City, UT 84132
Phone: (801) 581-7201

Fax: (801) 585-3300
E-mail: deans.admissions@hsc.utah.edu
http://www.med.utah.edu/som/
Application: AMCAS
Deadline: October 15
Type of School: Public

Vermont

UNIVERSITY OF VERMONT

College of Medicine
Admissions Office
C-225 Given Bldg.
Burlington, VT 05405
Phone: (802) 656-2154
http://www.med.uvm.edu/
Application: AMCAS
Deadline: November 1
Type of School: Public

Virginia

EASTERN VIRGINIA MEDICAL SCHOOL

Office of Admissions
P.O. Box 1980
Norfolk, VA 23501
Phone: (757) 446-5812
Fax: (757) 446-5896
http://www.evms.edu/
Application: AMCAS
Deadline: November 15
Type of School: Private

UNIVERSITY OF VIRGINIA

Admissions Office
School of Medicine, # 235
Charlottesville, VA 22908
Phone: (804) 924-5571
Fax: (804) 982-2586
E-mail: bab7g@virginia.edu
http://www.med.virginia.edu/schools/medschl.html
Application: AMCAS
Deadline: November 1
Type of School: Public

VIRGINIA COMMONWEALTH UNIVERSITY

Medical College of Virginia Campus
School of Medicine
Medical School Admissions
MCV Station Box 980565
Richmond, VA 23298-0565
Phone: (804) 828-9629
Fax: (804) 828-1246
http://www.medschool.vcu.edu/
Application: AMCAS
Deadline: November 15
Type of School: Public

Washington

UNIVERSITY OF WASHINGTON

School of Medicine
Office of Admissions
A-300 Health Sciences Center
Box 356340
Seattle, WA 98195-6340
Phone: (206) 543-7212
E-mail: askuwsom@u.washington.edu
http://www.washington.edu/medical/som/
Application: AMCAS
Deadline: November 1
Type of School: Public

West Virginia

MARSHALL UNIVERSITY

School of Medicine
Admissions Office
1600 Medical Center Drive
Suite 3400
Huntington, WV 25701
Phone: (304) 691-1738
Fax: (304) 691-1740
http://musom.marshall.edu/
Application: AMCAS
Deadline: November 15
Type of School: Public

APPENDIX A

WEST VIRGINIA UNIVERSITY

School of Medicine
Office of Admissions and Records
Health Sciences Center
P.O. Box 9815
Morgantown, WV 26506
Phone: (304) 293-3521
E-mail: eluzader@mail.arc.wvu.edu
http://www.hsc.wvu.edu/som/md.htm
Application: AMCAS
Deadline: November 15
Type of School: Public

Wisconsin

MEDICAL COLLEGE OF WISCONSIN

Office of Admissions and Registrar
8701 Watertown Plank Road
Milwaukee, WI 53226
Phone: (414) 456-8296
Fax: (414) 456-6506
http://www.mcw.edu/
Application: AMCAS
Deadline: November 1
Type of School: Private

UNIVERSITY OF WISCONSIN MEDICAL SCHOOL

Admissions Committee
Medical Sciences Center, Room 1140
1300 University Avenue
Madison, WI 53706-1532
Phone: (608) 263-4925
Fax: (608) 262-2327
http://www.medsch.wisc.edu/index.html
Application: AMCAS
Deadline: October 15
Type of School: Public

CANADA

Alberta

UNIVERSITY OF ALBERTA

Faculty of Medicine and Dentistry
Admissions Office
2-45 Medical Sciences Building
Edmonton, Alberta
Canada T6G 2H7
Phone: (780) 492-6350
E-mail: admission@med.ualberta.ca
http://www.med.ualberta.ca/
Deadline: November 1
*Does not accept foreign students.

UNIVERSITY OF CALGARY

Faculty of Medicine
Office of Admissions
3330 Hospital Drive, NW
Calgary, Alberta
Canada T2N 4N1
Phone: (403) 220-6849
Fax: (403) 283-4740
E-mail: meyers@med.ucalgary.ca
http://www.med.ucalgary.ca/
Deadline: November 15

British Columbia

UNIVERSITY OF BRITISH COLUMBIA

Faculty of Medicine
Office of the Dean, Admissions Office
317-2194 Health Sciences Mall
Vancouver, British Columbia
Canada V6T 1Z3
Phone: (604) 822-4482
E-mail: admissions.md@ubc.ca
http://www.med.ubc.ca/education.htm
Deadline: December 1

Manitoba

UNIVERSITY OF MANITOBA

Faculty of Medicine, Registrar
S 204 – 753 McDermot Avenue
Winnipeg, Manitoba
Canada R3E 0W3
Phone: (204) 789-3499
Fax: (204) 789-3929
http://www.umanitoba.ca/faculties/
medicine/admissions/index.html
Deadline: November 15

Newfoundland

MEMORIAL UNIVERSITY OF NEWFOUNDLAND

Faculty of Medicine
Admissions Office
Room 1751, Health Sciences Centre
St. John's, NF
Canada A1B 3V6
Phone: (709) 737-6615
Fax: (709) 737-5186
E-mail: munmed@morgan.ucs.mun.ca
http://www.med.mun.ca/med/admissio
Deadline: November 15

Nova Scotia

DALHOUSIE UNIVERSITY

Faculty of Medicine
Admissions Coordinator
Room C-132, Lower Level
Clinical Research Centre
5849 University Avenue
Halifax, NS
Canada B3H 4H7
Phone: (902) 494-1083
Fax: (902) 494-8884
http://www.medicine.dal.ca/
Deadline: November 15

Ontario

MCMASTER UNIVERSITY

Faculty of Health Sciences
M.D. Admissions and Records
Health Sciences Center Room 1B7
1200 Main Street West
Hamilton, Ontario
Canada L8N 3Z5
Phone: (905) 525-9140 ext. 22235
E-mail: mdadmit@fhs.csu.mcmaster.ca
http://www-fhs.mcmaster.ca/
Application: OMSAS
Deadline: October 15

QUEEN'S UNIVERSITY

Faculty of Medicine
Admissions Office
Kingston, Ontario
Canada K7L 3N6
Phone: (613) 533-2542
Fax: (613) 533-6884
E-mail: jeb8@post.queensu.ca
http://meds.queensu.ca/medicine/
Application: OMSAS
Deadline: October 15

UNIVERSITY OF OTTAWA

Faculty of Medicine
Admissions, 451 Smyth Road
Ottawa, Ontario
Canada K1H 8M5
Phone: (613) 562-5409
Fax: (613) 562-5420
E-mail: nracine@uottowa.ca
Application: OMSAS
http://www.uottawa.ca/academic/med/
Deadline: October 15

UNIVERSITY OF TORONTO

Faculty of Medicine
Admissions Office
1 Kings College Circle
Toronto, Ontario
Canada M5S 1A8

Phone: (416) 978-6585
E-mail: medicine.web@utoronto.ca
http://www.library.utoronto.ca/medicine/
Application: OMSAS
Deadline: October 15

UNIVERSITY OF WESTERN ONTARIO

Faculty of Medicine and Dentistry
Admissions Office
Medical Sciences Building
Room M-103
London, Ontario
Canada N6A 5C1
Phone: (519) 661-3744
Fax: (519) 661-3797
E-mail: admissions@med.uwo.ca
http://www.med.uwo.ca/
Application: OMSAS
Deadline: October 15

Quebec

UNIVERSITÉ LAVAL

Faculty of Medicine
Admissions Committee
Ste-Foy, Quebec
Canada G1K 7P4
Phone: (418) 656-2131, Ext. 2492
E-mail: admission@fmed.ulaval.ca
http://www.fmed.ulaval.ca/
Deadlines: March 1 (Canadians), February 1 (non-Canadians)

MCGILL UNIVERSITY

Faculty of Medicine
Admissions Office
3655 Drummond Street
Montreal, Quebec
Canada H3G 1Y6
Phone: (514) 398-3517
Fax: (514) 398-4631
E-mail: medadm@medcor.mcgill.ca
http://www.med.mcgill.ca/
Deadlines: November 15 (out of province), January 15 (Quebec resident applicants to 4 year program), March 1 (Quebec resident applicants to 5-year program)

UNIVERSITY OF MONTREAL

Faculty of Medicine
Committee on Admission
PO Box 6128, Station Centre-Ville
Montreal, Quebec
Canada H3C 3J7
Phone: (514) 343-6265
E-mail: admmed@ere.umontreal.ca
http://www.med.umontreal.ca/
Deadline: March 1

UNIVERSITY OF SHERBROOKE

Faculty of Medicine
Admission Office
3001 12th Avenue
Sherbrooke, Quebec
Canada J1H 5N4
Phone: (819) 564-5208
Fax: (819) 564-5378
E-mail: admmed@courrier.usherb.ca
http://www.usherb.ca/
Deadline: March 1

Saskatchewan

UNIVERSITY OF SASKATCHEWAN

College of Medicine
Secretary, Admissions
B103 Health Sciences Building
Saskatoon, Saskatchewan
Canada S7N 5E5
Phone: (306) 966-8554
Fax: (306) 966-6164
E-mail: lobergh@admin.usask.ca
http://www.usask.ca/medicine/index.html
Deadlines: December 1 (out of province), January 15 (in province)

Osteopathic Medical Schools

ARIZONA COLLEGE OF OSTEOPATHIC MEDICINE—A COLLEGE OF MIDWESTERN UNIVERSITY (AZCOM)

Office of Admissions
19555 N. 59th Avenue
Glendale, Arizona 85308
Phone: (602) 572-3215
http://www.midwestern.edu/
Pages/AZCOM.html

CHICAGO COLLEGE OF OSTEOPATHIC MEDICINE—A COLLEGE OF MIDWESTERN UNIVERSITY (CCOM)

Admissions Office
555 31st Street
Downers Grove, Illinois 60515-1235
Phone: (630) 969-4400
Fax: (630) 971-6086
http://www.midwestern.edu/
Pages/CCOM.html

KIRKSVILLE COLLEGE OF OSTEOPATHIC MEDICINE (KCOM)

Admissions Office
800 West Jefferson Street
Kirksville, Missouri 63501
Phone: (660) 626-2237
Fax: (660) 626-2969
E-mail: admissions@fileserver7.kcom.edu
http://www.kcom.edu/

LAKE ERIE COLLEGE OF OSTEOPATHIC MEDICINE (LECOM)

Office of Admissions
1858 W. Grandview Boulevard
Erie, Pennsylvania 16509
Phone: (814) 866-6641
Fax: (814) 866-8123
http://www.lecom.edu

MICHIGAN STATE UNIVERSITY COLLEGE OF OSTEOPATHIC MEDICINE (MSU-COM)

Director of Admissions
C110 East Fee Hall
East Lansing, Michigan 48824
Phone: (517) 353-7740
http://www.com.msu.edu

NEW YORK COLLEGE OF OSTEOPATHIC MEDICINE OF NEW YORK INSTITUTE OF TECHNOLOGY (NYCOM)

Director of Admissions
Wheatley Road, Box 8000
Old Westbury, New York 11568
Phone: (516) 626-6900
Fax: (516) 686-3831
http://www.nyit.edu/NYCOM/

NOVA SOUTHEASTERN UNIVERSITY COLLEGE OF OSTEOPATHIC MEDICINE (NSUCOM)

Admissions Office
3200 S. University Drive
Fort Lauderdale, Florida 33328
Phone: (954) 262-1126
Fax: (954) 262-2282
E-mail: rogeria@hpd.nova.edu
http://medicine.nova.edu

OHIO UNIVERSITY COLLEGE OF OSTEOPATHIC MEDICINE (OUCOM)

Office of Admissions
102 Grosvenor Hall
Athens, Ohio 45701-2979
Phone: (800) 345-1560
Fax: (740) 593-2256
E-mail: Admissions@exchange.oucom.ohiou.edu
http://www.oucom.ohiou.edu/

OKLAHOMA STATE UNIVERSITY COLLEGE OF OSTEOPATHIC MEDICINE (OSU/COM)

Admissions Office
1111 West 17th Street
Tulsa, Oklahoma 74107
Phone: (800) 677-1972
Fax: (918) 561-8250
http://osu.com.okstate.edu/osucom.html

PHILADELPHIA COLLEGE OF OSTEOPATHIC MEDICINE (PCOM)

Admissions Office
4170 City Avenue
Philadelphia, Pennsylvania 19131
Phone: (215) 871-6701
Fax: (215) 871-6719
E-mail: admissions@pcom.edu
http://www.pcom.edu

PIKEVILLE COLLEGE SCHOOL OF OSTEOPATHIC MEDICINE (PCSOM)

Admissions Office
214 Sycamore Street
Pikeville, KY 41501-1194
Phone: (606) 432-9617
Fax: (606) 432-9669
E-mail: klwmson@pc.edu
http://www.pc.edu

TOURO UNIVERSITY COLLEGE OF OSTEOPATHIC MEDICINE (TUCOM)

832 Walnut Street
Quarters C
Vallejo, CA 94592
Phone: (707) 638-5270
Fax: (707) 638-5250
E-mail: haight@adminm.touro.edu
http://tucom.edu

THE UNIVERSITY OF HEALTH SCIENCES— COLLEGE OF OSTEOPATHIC MEDICINE (UHS-COM)

Office of Admissions
1750 Independence Boulevard
Kansas City, Missouri 64106-1453
Phone: (800) 234-4UHS
Fax: (816) 283-2349
http://www.uhs.edu

UNIVERSITY OF MEDICINE AND DENTISTRY OF NEW JERSEY SCHOOL OF OSTEOPATHIC MEDICINE (UMDNJ-SOM)

Office of Admissions
One Medical Center Drive, Suite 162
Stratford, New Jersey 08084-1504
Phone: (856) 566-7050
Fax: (856) 566-6895
E-mail: somadm@umdnj.edu
http://www3.umdnj.edu/som/index.html

UNIVERSITY OF NEW ENGLAND COLLEGE OF OSTEOPATHIC MEDICINE (UNECOM)

Admissions Office
11 Hills Beach Road
Biddeford, Maine 04005
Phone: (207) 283-0171
Fax: (207) 294-5908
http://www.une.edu/COM/compage1.html

UNIVERSITY OF NORTH TEXAS HEALTH SCIENCE CENTER—TEXAS COLLEGE OF OSTEOPATHIC MEDICINE (UNTHSC)

Office of Medical Student Admissions
3500 Camp Bowie Boulevard
Fort Worth, Texas 76107-2699
Phone: (800) 535-TCOM
Fax: (817) 735-2225
E-mail: TCOMAdmissions@hsc.unt.edu
http://www.hsc.unt.edu/education/tcom/admis.html

UNIVERSITY OF OSTEOPATHIC MEDICINE AND HEALTH SCIENCES—COLLEGE OF OSTEOPATHIC MEDICINE AND SURGERY (UOMHS/COMS)

Director of Admissions and Financial Aid
3200 Grand Avenue
Des Moines, Iowa 50312
Phone: (515) 271-1450
Fax: (515) 271-1578
E-mail: doadmit@dsmu.edu
http://www.uomhs.edu

WEST VIRGINIA SCHOOL OF OSTEOPATHIC MEDICINE (WVSOM)

Director of Admissions
400 North Lee Street
Lewisburg, West Virginia 24901
Phone: (800) 35-OSTEO
Fax: (304) 645-4859
E-mail: warren@mail.osteo.wvnet.edu
http://www.wvsom.edu

WESTERN UNIVERSITY OF THE HEALTH SCIENCES—COLLEGE OF OSTEOPATHIC MEDICINE OF THE PACIFIC (WesternU/COMP)

309 East Second Street
College Plaza
Pomona, California 91766-1854
Phone: (909) 469-5335
Fax: (909) 469-5570
E-mail: admissions@westernu.edu
http://www.westernu.edu/comp.html

How Did We Do? Grade Us.

Thank you for choosing a Kaplan book. Your comments and suggestions are very useful to us. Please answer the following questions to assist us in our continued development of high-quality resources to meet your needs.

The Kaplan book I read was: _____

My name is: _____

My address is: _____

_____

My e-mail address is: _____

What overall grade would you give this book?   (A) (B) (C) (D) (F)

How relevant was the information to your goals?   (A) (B) (C) (D) (F)

How comprehensive was the information in this book?   (A) (B) (C) (D) (F)

How accurate was the information in this book?   (A) (B) (C) (D) (F)

How easy was the book to use?   (A) (B) (C) (D) (F)

How appealing was the book's design?   (A) (B) (C) (D) (F)

What were the book's strong points? _____

How could this book be improved? _____

Is there anything that we left out that you wanted to know more about?

Would you recommend this book to others?   ☐ YES   ☐ NO

Other comments: _____

_____

_____

Do we have permission to quote you?   ☐ YES   ☐ NO

Thank you for your help. Please tear out this page and mail it to:

Dave Chipps, Managing Editor
Kaplan Educational Centers
888 Seventh Avenue
New York, NY 10106

Or, you can submit your comments electronically by using Kaplan's online feedback form at http://www.kaptest.com/customer-service/lvl5_comments.jhtml

Thanks!

SIXTY · YEARS · OF
KAPLAN
60
BUILDING · FUTURES

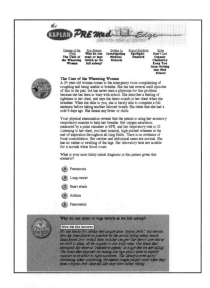
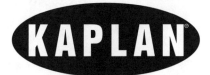

About

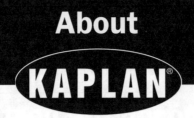

Kaplan, Inc. is one of the nation's leading providers of education and career services. Kaplan is a wholly owned subsidiary of The Washington Post Company.

KAPLAN TEST PREPARATION & ADMISSIONS

Kaplan's nationally recognized test prep courses cover more than 20 standardized tests, including secondary school, college and graduate school entrance exams, as well as foreign language and professional licensing exams. In addition, Kaplan offers a college admissions course, private tutoring, and a variety of free information and services for students applying to college and graduate programs. Kaplan also provides information and guidance on the financial aid process. Students can enroll in online test prep courses and admissions consulting services at www.kaptest.com.

Kaplan K12 Learning Services partners with schools, universities, and teachers to help students succeed, providing customized assessment, education, and professional development programs.

SCORE! EDUCATIONAL CENTERS

SCORE! after-school learning centers help K–10 students build confidence along with academic skills in a motivating, sports-oriented environment.

SCORE! Prep provides in-home, one-on-one tutoring for high school academic subjects and standardized tests.

eSCORE.com is the first educational services Web site to offer parents and kids newborn to age 18 personalized child development and educational resources online.

KAPLANCOLLEGE.COM

KaplanCollege.com, Kaplan's distance learning platform, offers an array of online educational programs for working professionals who want to advance their careers. Learners will find nearly 500 professional development, continuing education, certification, and degree courses and programs in Nursing, Education, Criminal Justice, Real Estate, Legal Professions, Law, Management, General Business, and Computing/Information Technology.

KAPLAN PUBLISHING

Kaplan Publishing produces retail books and software. Kaplan Books, published by Simon & Schuster, include titles in test preparation, admissions, education, career development, and life skills; Kaplan and *Newsweek* jointly publish guides on getting into college, finding the right career, and helping children succeed in school.

KAPLAN PROFESSIONAL

Kaplan Professional provides assessment, training, and certification services for corporate clients and individuals seeking to advance their careers. Member units include:

- Dearborn, a leading supplier of licensing training and continuing education for securities, real estate, and insurance professionals

- Perfect Access/CRN, which delivers software education and consultation for law firms and businesses

- Kaplan Professional Call Center Services, a total provider of services for the call center industry

- Self Test Software, a world leader in exam simulation software and preparation for technical certifications

- Schweser's Study Program/AIAF, which provides preparation services for the CFA examination

KAPLAN INTERNATIONAL PROGRAMS

Kaplan assists international students and professionals in the United States through a series of intensive English language and test preparation programs. These programs are offered at campus-based centers across the United States. Specialized services include housing, placement at top American universities, fellowship management, academic monitoring and reporting, and financial administration.

COMMUNITY OUTREACH

Kaplan provides educational career resources to thousands of financially disadvantaged students annually, working closely with educational institutions, not-for-profit groups, government agencies and grass roots organizations on a variety of national and local support programs. These programs help students and professionals from a variety of backgrounds achieve their educational and career goals.

BRASSRING

BrassRing Inc., the premier business-to-business hiring management and recruitment services company, offers employers a vertically integrated suite of online and offline solutions. BrassRing, created in September 1999, combined Kaplan Career Services, Terra-Starr, Crimson & Brown Associates, thepavement.com, and HireSystems. In March 2000, BrassRing acquired Career Service Inc./Westech. Kaplan is a shareholder in BrassRing, along with Tribune Company, Central Newspapers, and Accel Partners.

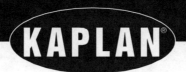

Want more information about our services, products, or the nearest Kaplan center?

1 Call our nationwide toll-free numbers:

1-800-KAP-TEST for information on our courses, private tutoring and admissions consulting

1-800-KAP-ITEM for information on our books and software

2 Connect with us in cyberspace:

On AOL, keyword:"Kaplan"

On the World Wide Web, go to:

1. www.kaplan.com
2. www.kaptest.com
3. www.eSCORE.com
4. www.dearborn.com
5. www.BrassRing.com
6. www.concordlawschool.com
7. www.KaplanCollege.com

Via e-mail: info@kaplan.com

3 Write to:

Kaplan, Inc.
888 Seventh Avenue
New York, NY 10106

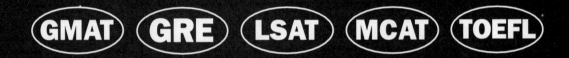
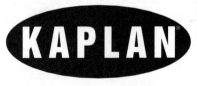